The AYURVEDA Home Cure Handbook

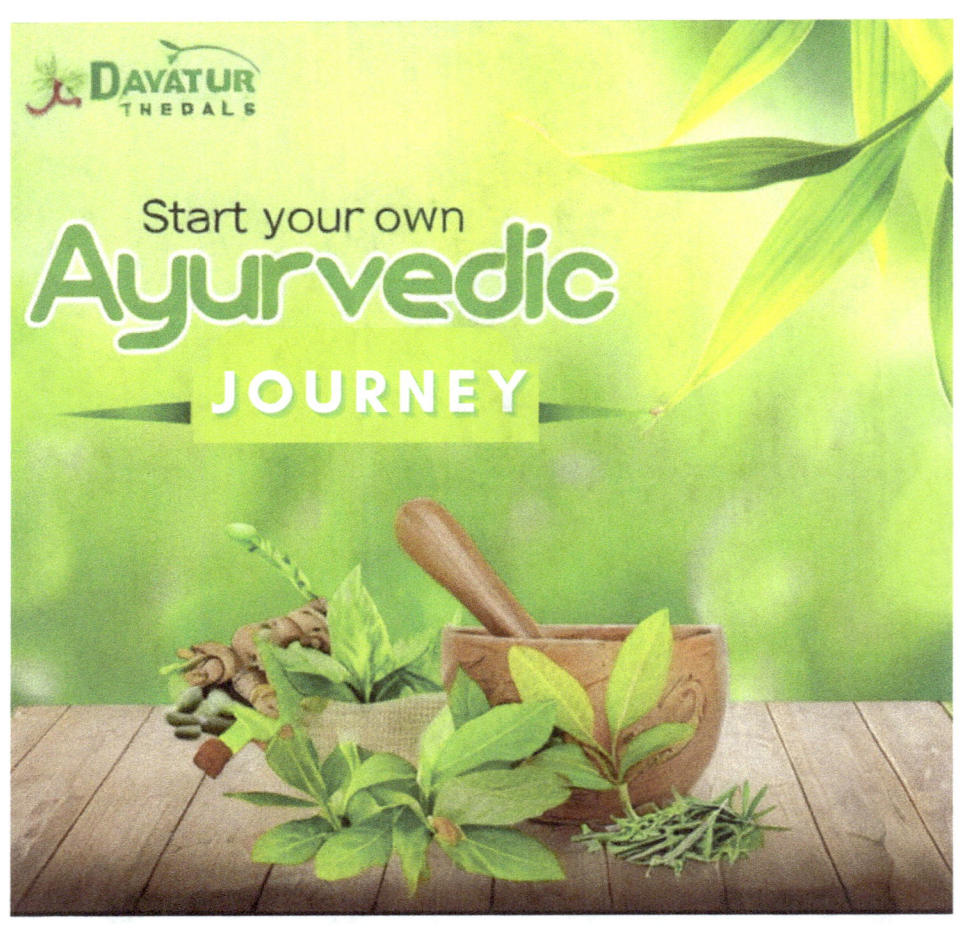

" Natural Home Healing Remedies"

DISCRIPTION

"The Ayurveda Home Cure Handbook" offers a life-changing path to improved health. This extensive manual is your key to the knowledge of Ayurveda, the age-old holistic healing discipline, and a happier, more balanced existence.

Interest: Discover the mysteries of natural healing and take charge of your health with simple-to-follow solutions. With a plethora of Ayurveda remedies for anything from common illnesses to everyday self-care routines, this guide will improve your health.

Desire: Picture a world in which common health issues can be resolved using items found in your kitchen. Explore a wealth of Ayurveda practices, rituals, and foods that can help you feel better physically, mentally, and spiritually.

Take action by assuming responsibility for your health and starting a self-care regimen. "The Ayurveda Home Cure Handbook" gives you the useful tools you need to incorporate Ayurveda principles into your daily life for a balanced and vibrant life.

Result: Feel the profound effects of Ayurveda on your general health. With the advice in these critical pages, you can bid stress a fond farewell, welcome vitality, and develop a life of holistic health. This is where your path to a better life begins.

Take action by assuming responsibility for your health and starting a self-care regimen. "The Ayurveda Home Cure Handbook" gives you the useful tools you need to incorporate Ayurvedic principles into your daily life for a balanced and vibrant life.

Result: Feel the profound effects of Ayurveda on your general health. With the advice in these critical pages, you can bid stress a fond farewell, welcome vitality, and develop a life of holistic health. This is where your path to a better life begins.

This manual is your go-to source for embracing Ayurveda at home and guaranteeing a life of sustained well-being, regardless of your level of experience.

INDEX

1. Turmeric (Haldi): 1~4
2. Ginger (Adrak): 5~8
3. Cumin (Jeera): 9~12
4. Coriander (Dhania): 13~15
5. Fennel (Saunf): 16~19
6. Tulsi (Holy Basil): 20~24
7. Amla (Indian Gooseberry): 25~27
8. Neem: 28~31
9. Ashwagandha: 32~35
10. Triphala: 36~40
11. Ghee: 41~44
12. Cardamom (Elaichi): 45~47
13. Ajwain (Carom Seeds): 48~51
14. Lemon (Nimbu): 52~54
15. Sesame Oil (Til Tel): 55~57
16. Castor Oil (Arandi Tel): 58~61
17. Trikatu Churna: 62~65
18. Brahmi: 66~69
19. Shatavari: 70~73
20. Guduchi (Giloy): 74~77

21. Mulethi (Licorice): 78~81
22. Haritaki: 82~86
23. Bhringraj Oil: 87~90
24. Gotu Kola (Mandukaparni): 91~94
25. Aloe Vera: 95~98
26. Arjuna: 99~102
27. Trikatu Churna: 103~106
28. Dandelion Tea: 107~110
29. Pippali (Long Pepper): 111~114
30. Kutki: 115~118
31. Bilva (Bael): 119~122
32. Kalmegh: 123~126
33. Mustard Oil (Sarson Tel): 127~130
34. Kesar (Saffron): 131~134
35. Manjistha: 135~138
36. Chyawanprash: 139~142
37. Gokshura: 143~146
38. Bamboo Rice: 147~150
39. Shankhpushpi: 151~154
40. Punarva: 155~158
41. Vacha (Sweet Flag): 159~162
42. Khadira: 163~166

43. Bael Juice:　　　　　　　　　　167~170
44. Kokum:　　　　　　　　　　　171~174
45. Jatamansi:　　　　　　　　　 176~179
46. Dashmool:　　　　　　　　　 180~184
47. Kumari (Aloe Vera Juice):　　　185~187
48. Yastimadhu (Licorice):　　　　188~191
49. Vidari Kanda:　　　　　　　　192~195
50. Punarnava:　　　　　　　　　196~200

TURMERIC (HALDI)

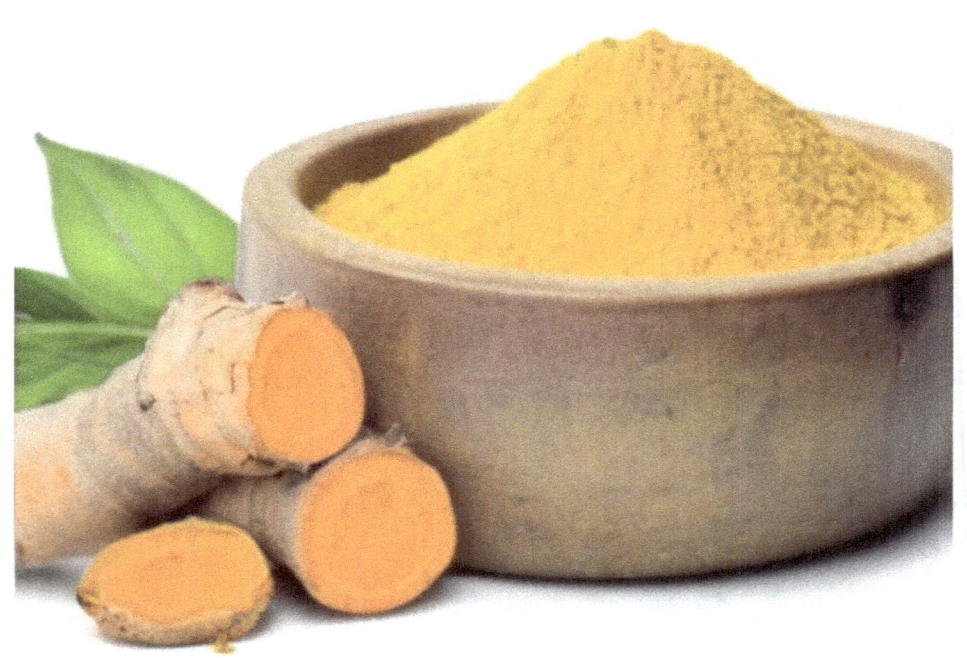

Anti-inflammatory and antioxidant properties.

Turmeric has been used for centuries in traditional medicine, particularly in South Asian countries. It is widely known for its culinary uses, giving a warm and slightly bitter flavor to dishes. Additionally, turmeric has been valued for its potential health benefits due to its anti-inflammatory, antioxidant, and antimicrobial properties.

1. **Properties of Turmeric:**

Curcumin Content: The primary active component of turmeric is a molecule known as curcumin. The anti-inflammatory, antioxidant, and anticancer effects of curcumin are well recognized.

Strong antioxidant qualities found in turmeric aid in the body's defence against free radicals. Oxidative stress brought on by free radicals can harm cells and have a role in a number of illnesses.

Anti-Inflammatory: Curcumin's anti-inflammatory properties have been investigated; these properties may be useful in the treatment of inflammatory illnesses such inflammatory bowel disease and arthritis.

Antiviral and Antibacterial: The antiviral and antibacterial qualities of turmeric can support the health of the immune system as a whole.

2. **Benefits of Turmeric:**

Anti-Inflammatory Effects: By lowering inflammation in the body, turmeric may be able to lessen the symptoms of arthritic disorders.

Benefits of Antioxidants: Turmeric's antioxidants may help shield the body from oxidative stress and may be involved in the prevention of chronic illnesses.

Digestive Health: Turmeric is believed to support digestive health by promoting the production of digestive enzymes and reducing inflammation in the digestive tract.

Joint Health: Some studies suggest that turmeric may help manage symptoms of osteoarthritis and rheumatoid arthritis due to its anti-inflammatory effects.

Heart Health: Curcumin has been studied for its potential benefits in reducing the risk of heart disease by improving the function of the endothelium (the lining of blood vessels) and lowering levels of inflammation and oxidation.

GINGER (ADRAK)

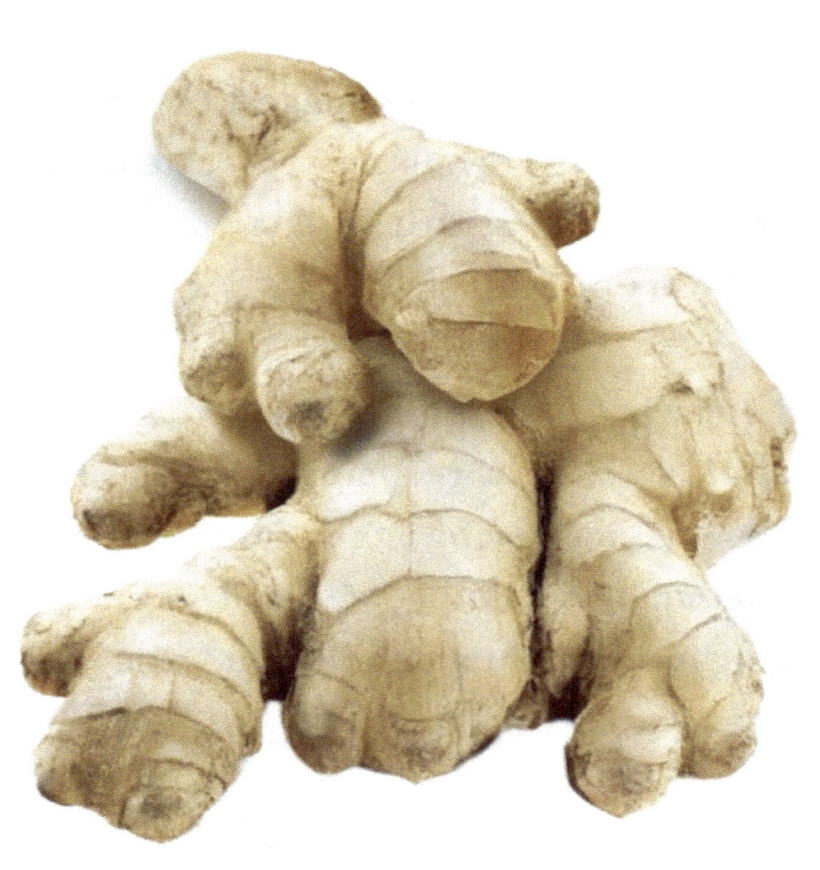

Aids digestion and reduces nausea.

A flowering plant with an underground stem known as a rhizome, ginger is used both medicinally and as a spice. Zingiber officinale is the plant's scientific name. The portion of the plant utilised for cooking and its possible medicinal properties is called the rhizome, or ginger root.

Important qualities of ginger include:

Ginger has a unique flavor that is strong, spicy, and slightly sweet. It gives a variety of foods richness and warmth.

Look: The ginger plant has a maximum height of three feet. The flowers are yellow-green with purple lips, while the leaves are long and slender and green.

Rhizome: The portion of the ginger plant that is harvested for food is the rhizome. Its exterior layer is strong and its colour is beige or yellowish.

Ginger's Health Benefits:

Anti-Nausea: Ginger is a well-known medicine for motion sickness, morning sickness during pregnancy, and nausea related to chemotherapy because of its capacity to reduce nausea and vomiting.

Anti-Inflammatory: Bioactive chemicals found in ginger have anti-inflammatory qualities that may aid in the body's natural reduction of inflammation.

Digestive Health: Ginger has been used to ease gastrointestinal pain and promote better digestion. It might relieve bloating and reflux.

Analgesic (pain-relieving) properties: Studies have indicated that ginger may be useful in controlling specific forms of pain, such as pain associated with osteoarthritis.

Immune System Support: Ginger's antioxidants may help maintain the general health of the immune system.

CUMIN (JEERA)

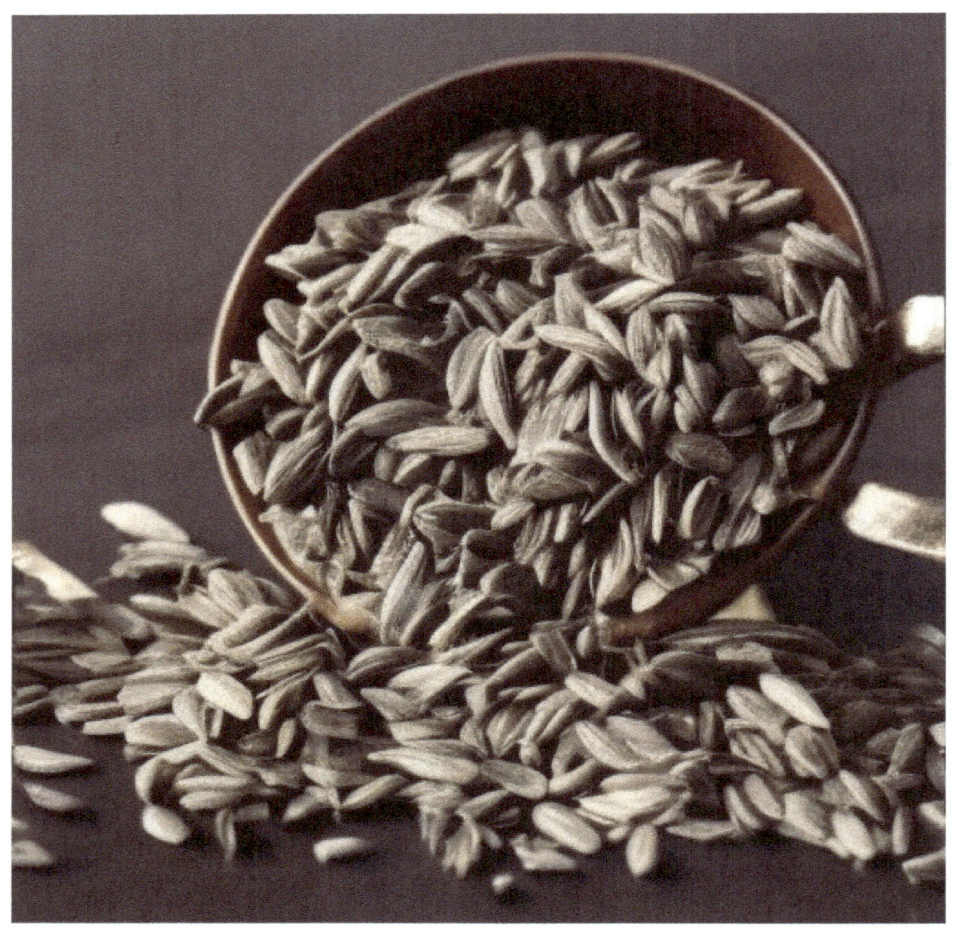

Improves digestion and metabolism.

Properties:

1. Flavor: Cumin has a warm, earthy, and slightly nutty flavor.
2. Aroma: The seeds release a strong aroma when toasted or ground.
3. Common Use: It is a key ingredient in many cuisines, particularly in Indian, Middle Eastern, and Mexican cooking.

Health Benefits of Cumin:

Digestive Health: The digestive qualities of cumin are well-known. It may lessen indigestion symptoms and help to stimulate the synthesis of digestive enzymes.

Anti-Inflammatory: The anti-inflammatory chemicals in cumin may aid in the body's reduction of inflammation.

Antioxidant-Rich: The seeds have a lot of antioxidants that can help fight off free radicals and shield cells from harm.

Weight Management: Research indicates that cumin may help manage weight by decreasing body fat and encouraging weight reduction.

Iron Absorption: For those who suffer from iron-deficiency anaemia, cumin may improve the body's ability to absorb iron from food.

Anti-Diabetic Properties: Some research indicates that cumin may help lower blood sugar levels, which may be advantageous for those who have diabetes.

Antimicrobial Effects: Studies on cumin have revealed antimicrobial qualities that may aid in the prevention and treatment of illnesses.

Health of the Respiratory System: Cumin has been used traditionally in medicine to treat respiratory disorders like bronchitis and asthma.

Although cumin may offer a number of health benefits, it should only be used in a balanced diet and should never be used in place of competent medical advice or care. Furthermore, each person will react differently to spices and herbs, and some may be allergic or sensitive to particular ingredients.

Coriander (Dhania)

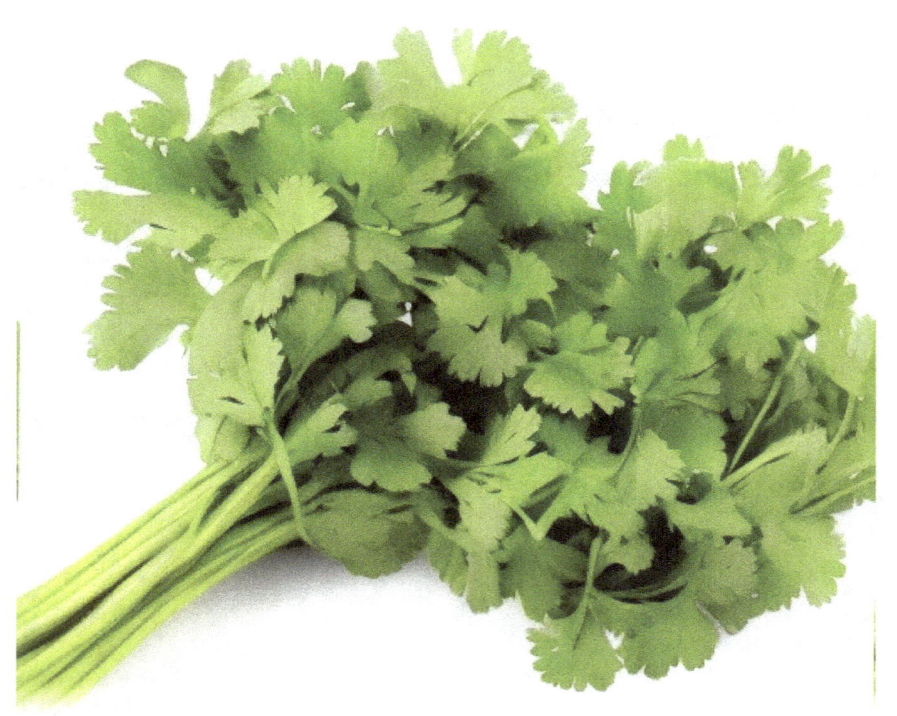

Detoxifies the body and aids digestion.

1. Herb and Spice:

- **Herb (Cilantro):** The leaves of the coriander plant are commonly used as an herb in many cuisines around the world. Cilantro has a fresh, citrusy flavor and is often used in salads, salsas, and as a garnish.
- **Spice (Coriander Seeds):** The seeds of the coriander plant are dried and used as a spice. Ground coriander is a common spice in various dishes, providing a warm and slightly citrusy flavor.

2. Nutritional Content:

Coriander is a good source of vitamins and minerals, including vitamin C, vitamin K, and potassium. It also contains antioxidants.

3. Health Benefits:

- **Digestive Health:** Coriander has been traditionally used to aid digestion and relieve gastrointestinal issues.

- **Antioxidant Properties:** The antioxidants in coriander may help combat oxidative stress and inflammation.
- **Blood Sugar Control:** Some studies suggest that coriander may have a positive impact on blood sugar levels.

4. Culinary Uses:

- Cilantro is a common ingredient in various cuisines, including Mexican, Indian, Middle Eastern, and Southeast Asian dishes.
- Coriander seeds are used in spice blends, pickling, and as a flavoring agent in both sweet and savory dishes.

5. Other Uses:

- Coriander is also used in traditional medicine and herbal remedies for various ailments.

Note: While many people enjoy the taste of coriander, there are some who have a genetic predisposition that makes cilantro taste soapy or unpleasant to them.

Fennel (Saunf)

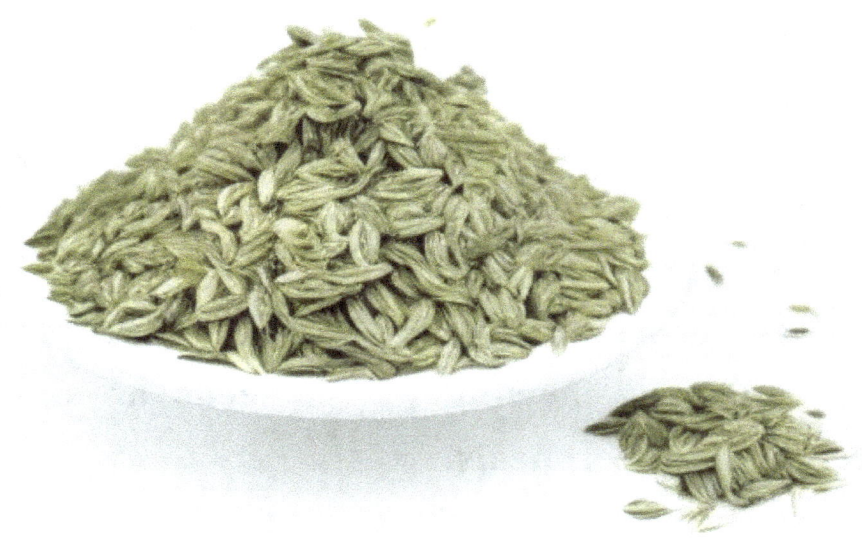

Eases digestion and freshens breath.

Fennel seeds are the dried seeds of the Foeniculum vulgare plant, which belongs to the carrot family. These seeds are commonly used as a spice in cooking and have a mild, sweet licorice-like flavor. Fennel seeds are often used in various culinary applications and traditional medicine due to their potential health benefits. Here are some of the benefits and uses of fennel seeds:

1. Digestive Aid: The digestive qualities of fennel seeds are well-known. They can aid in the relief of gas, bloating, and indigestion. Digestion may be aided by chewing fennel seeds or sipping fennel tea after meals.

2. Respiratory Health: Compounds in fennel seeds may help reduce respiratory problems and congestion. They are occasionally used to treat bronchitis symptoms and coughs.

3. Antioxidant Properties: Fennel seeds are rich in antioxidants, such as flavonoids, which may help protect the body's cells from damage caused by free radicals.

4. Anti-inflammatory Effects: Research indicates that fennel seeds may have anti-inflammatory qualities, which may help with inflammatory diseases.

5. Menstrual Health: It's thought that fennel seeds contain qualities that can lessen the discomfort associated with menstruation and help control menstrual cycles. Menstrual cramps are commonly treated with fennel tea.

6. Weight Management: Fennel seeds have few calories and have the potential to reduce hunger. By lessening the desire to overeat, fennel tea or seeds can aid with weight management.

7. Culinary Uses: Fennel seeds are used as a spice in various cuisines, especially in Indian, Mediterranean, and Middle Eastern dishes. They add a unique flavor to soups, stews, and curries.

8. Breath Freshener: Chewing fennel seeds can help freshen breath due to their aromatic and antibacterial properties.

9. Tea Infusion: A well-liked herbal cure is fennel seed tea. A straightforward infusion can be prepared by steeping crushed fennel seeds in boiling water. This tea is popular because it helps with digestion and promotes relaxation.

It's crucial to remember that while fennel seeds may have health benefits, everyone reacts differently. Before using fennel seeds in your diet or taking them as medicine, it's best to speak with a healthcare provider if you have any particular health issues.

Tulsi (Holy Basil)

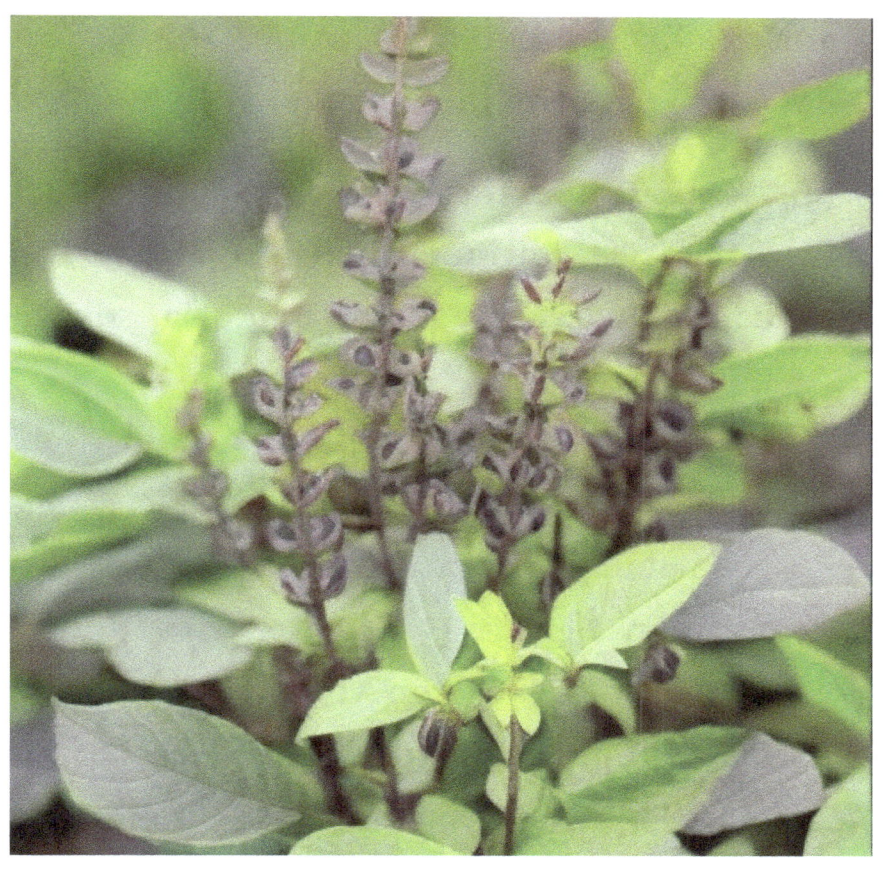

Boosts immunity and reduces stress.

Tulsi (Holy Basil):

- Benefits: Tulsi, also known as Holy Basil, is a sacred plant in Hinduism and is valued for its medicinal properties. It is rich in antioxidants and essential oils. Some potential benefits include:

1. Medicinal Properties:
   - Tulsi has antimicrobial properties that can help fight against bacteria, viruses, and fungi.
   - It has anti-inflammatory and anti-oxidative properties, which may contribute to overall health.
2. Respiratory Health:
   - Tulsi is known for its effectiveness in managing respiratory disorders. It may help alleviate symptoms of asthma, bronchitis, and other respiratory issues.

3. Stress Relief:
    - Tulsi is considered an adaptogen, which means it may help the body adapt to stress and normalize physiological functions.
4. Digestive Health:
    - It can aid digestion and help alleviate issues like indigestion and bloating.
5. Cardiovascular Health:
    - Some studies suggest that Tulsi may have a positive impact on heart health by reducing cholesterol levels and blood pressure.
6. Immune System Support:
    - Tulsi is believed to have immunomodulatory properties, helping to strengthen the immune system.

7. Skin Conditions:
    - Applied topically, Tulsi may help with skin conditions such as acne due to its antimicrobial and anti-inflammatory properties.
8. Traditional and Culinary Uses:
    - Tulsi is commonly used in traditional medicine systems like Ayurveda.
    - It is also used as a culinary herb in various dishes and teas.
9. Religious and Cultural Significance:
    - In Hinduism, Tulsi is considered a sacred plant and is often planted around homes. It is associated with various religious rituals and ceremonies.
10. Basil (Sweet Basil) Culinary Uses:
    - Basil, especially sweet basil, is popular in culinary applications. It is used in salads, pasta dishes, pesto, and various other recipes for its aromatic and flavorful leaves.

Remember that while these benefits are often supported by traditional use and some scientific studies, it's essential to consult with a healthcare professional for personalized advice, especially if you have specific health concerns or conditions.

Amla (Indian Gooseberry):

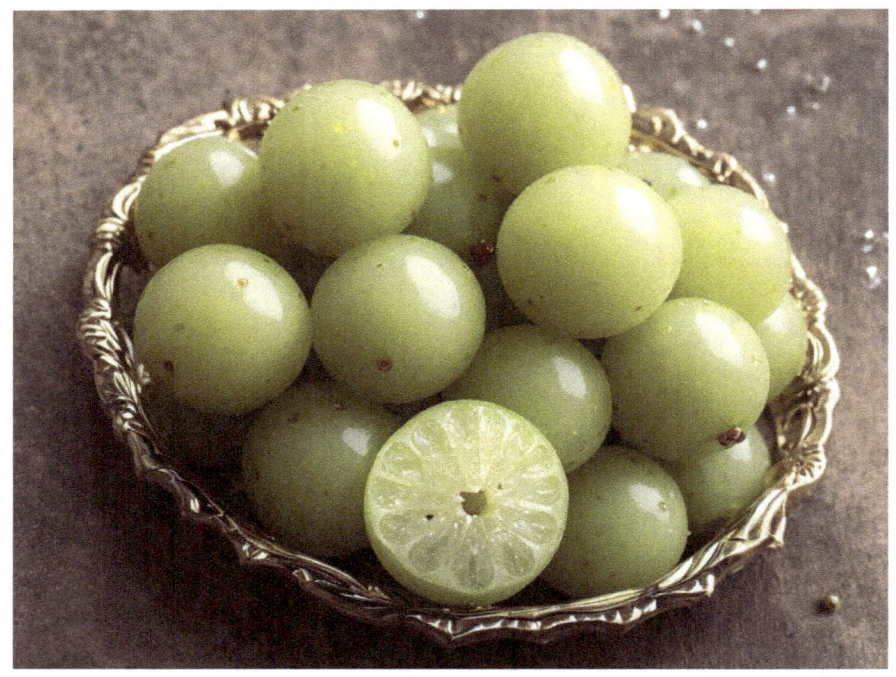

Amla (Indian Gooseberry): Rich in Vitamin C, strengthens the immune system.

Amla is rich in vitamin C, antioxidants, and other beneficial compounds. It is believed to have immunomodulatory, anti-inflammatory, and anti-aging properties. Some potential benefits of consuming Amla include:

1. Rich in Vitamin C: Amla is exceptionally high in vitamin C, which is essential for a healthy immune system, skin health, and overall well-being.
2. Antioxidant Properties: Amla is rich in antioxidants, which help combat oxidative stress in the body, reducing the risk of chronic diseases.
3. Digestive Health: Amla may aid in digestion and alleviate constipation. It is known to have a mild laxative effect.
4. Hair Health: Amla is often used in hair care products or as a hair mask due to its potential to strengthen hair, reduce hair loss, and promote hair growth.

5. **Cholesterol Regulation:** Research indicates that Amla could play a role in controlling cholesterol levels, which could have a positive impact on heart health.

6. **Blood Sugar Regulation:** Amla may help regulate blood sugar levels, according to some studies.

Amla can be taken in several ways, such as powder, juice, fresh fruit, or as a component of Ayurvedic remedies. Even while amla is generally seen to be safe, it's still a good idea to speak with a doctor before making any big dietary changes or using it for medical purposes, particularly if you have any underlying medical concerns or are taking medication.

Neem:

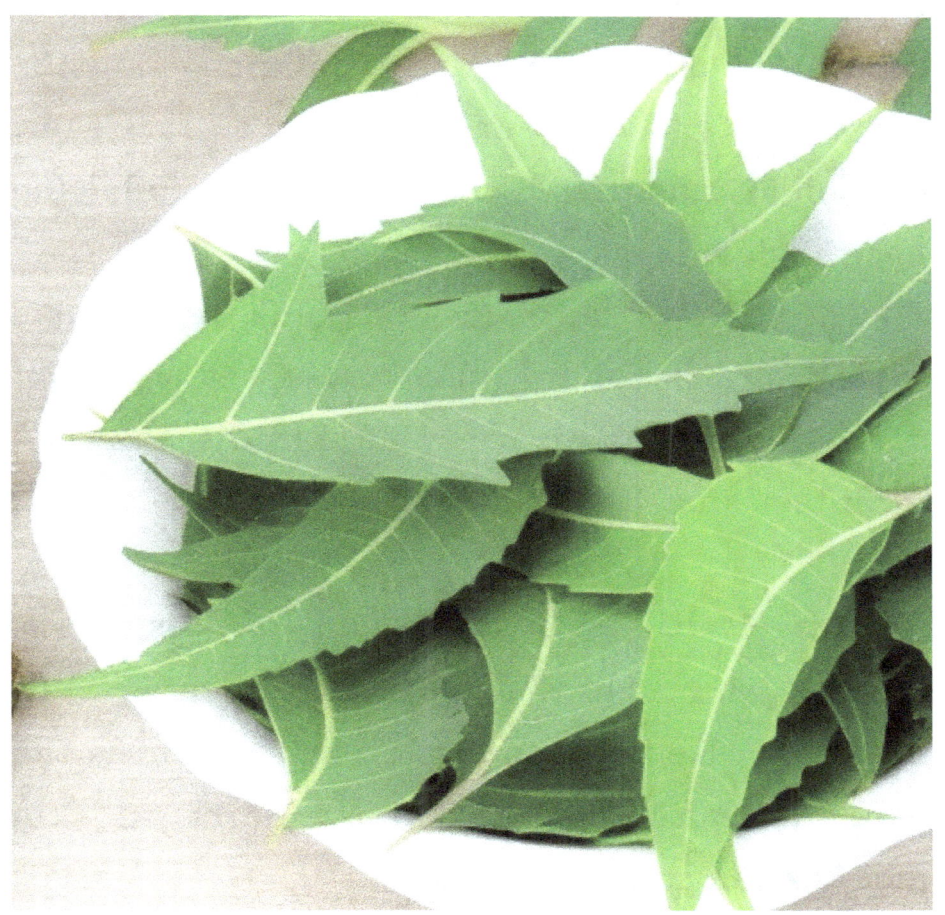

Antibacterial and anti fungal properties, supports skin health.

The Indian subcontinent is home to the neem tree, Azadirachta indica, which has long been utilized in traditional medicine. The leaves, bark, seeds, and oil of the neem tree are among the parts that have been recognized for their medicinal qualities. Neem has the following health advantages:

1. The strong antibacterial and anti-fungal characteristics of neem make it a useful treatment for a variety of skin diseases and infections.

2. Skin Health: Skin conditions like psoriasis, eczema, and acne are frequently treated with neem. It lessens inflammation and enhances the general health of the skin by aiding in skin purification and cleansing.

3. Dental Health: Neem is known for its use in dental care. It is used in traditional toothpaste and mouthwashes for its antibacterial properties, helping to prevent gum diseases and maintain oral hygiene.

4. **Immune System Support:** Neem is believed to have immune-boosting properties. Regular consumption or topical application may help support the body's natural defenses against infections.

5. **Anti-inflammatory Effects:** Neem has anti-inflammatory properties that may help in reducing inflammation and discomfort associated with various conditions.

6. **Blood Sugar Regulation:** Some studies suggest that neem may help in regulating blood sugar levels, making it potentially beneficial for individuals with diabetes.

7. **Antioxidant Properties:** Neem contains antioxidants that can help neutralize free radicals in the body, protecting cells from damage and supporting overall health.

8. **Insect Repellent:** Neem is a natural insect repellent. It is often used in the form of neem oil to repel mosquitoes and other insects.

9. **Anti-Cancer Properties:** Some research has explored neem's potential in inhibiting the growth of certain cancer cells, although more studies are needed to establish its efficacy in cancer treatment.

10. **Wound Healing:** Neem has been traditionally used for wound healing. Its antimicrobial and anti-inflammatory properties may help prevent infections and promote faster healing.

While neem offers numerous potential health benefits, it's important to note that more research is needed to fully understand its mechanisms and effectiveness in various applications. Additionally, individuals with specific medical conditions or allergies should consult with a healthcare professional before using neem products for therapeutic purposes.

Ashwagandha

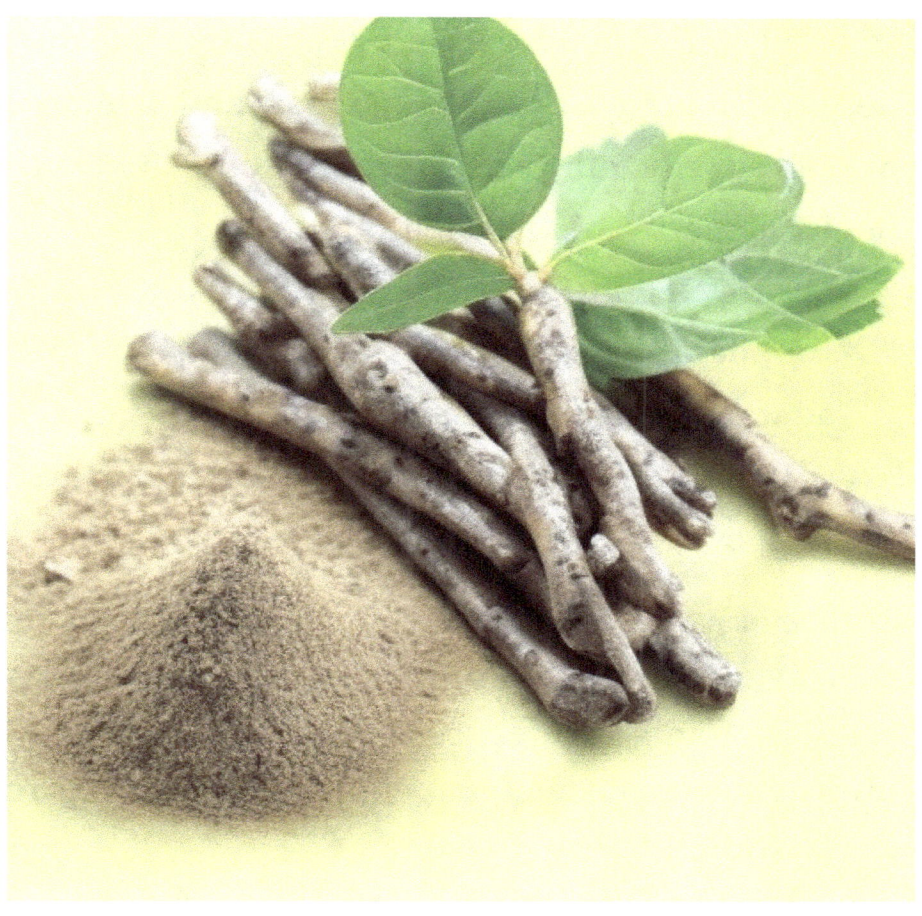

Adaptogenic herb, helps manage stress.

Ashwagandha, scientifically known as Withania somnifera, is an ancient medicinal herb that has been used in Ayurvedic medicine for centuries. It is classified as an adaptogen, which means it helps the body cope with stress and promotes overall well-being. Here are some potential health benefits of ashwagandha:

1. Stress Reduction: Ashwagandha is known for its adaptogenic properties, helping the body adapt to stress and promoting a sense of calmness. It may reduce cortisol levels, which are associated with stress.

2. Anxiety and Depression: Some studies suggest that ashwagandha may have anxiolytic (anxiety-reducing) and antidepressant effects, potentially improving symptoms in people with anxiety and depression.

3. Cognitive Function: There is evidence to suggest that ashwagandha may enhance cognitive function, including memory and attention. It may have neuroprotective effects that could be beneficial for brain health.

4. Anti-inflammatory Properties: Ashwagandha has been reported to have anti-inflammatory effects, which could be beneficial for conditions related to inflammation.

5. Immune System Support: Some studies indicate that ashwagandha may support the immune system, helping the body defend against infections and illnesses.

6. Energy and Vitality: Ashwagandha is believed to enhance energy levels and overall vitality, potentially reducing fatigue.

7. Hormonal Balance: It may have a positive impact on hormonal balance, particularly in managing cortisol levels, which can affect reproductive hormones and stress response.

8. Anti-Cancer Properties: While more research is needed, some studies suggest that ashwagandha may have anti-cancer properties by inhibiting the growth of certain types of cancer cells.

9. Blood Sugar Regulation: There is some evidence to suggest that ashwagandha may help regulate blood sugar levels, making it potentially beneficial for individuals with diabetes.

10. Heart Health: Ashwagandha may improve cholesterol and reduce blood pressure, among other cardiovascular benefits.

It is noteworthy that although ashwagandha exhibits potential benefits in a number of health domains, individual reactions may differ, and further investigation is required to completely comprehend its mechanisms and possible adverse effects. It is best to speak with a healthcare provider before using ashwagandha or any supplement in your regimen, particularly if you are taking medication or have pre-existing health conditions.

Triphala

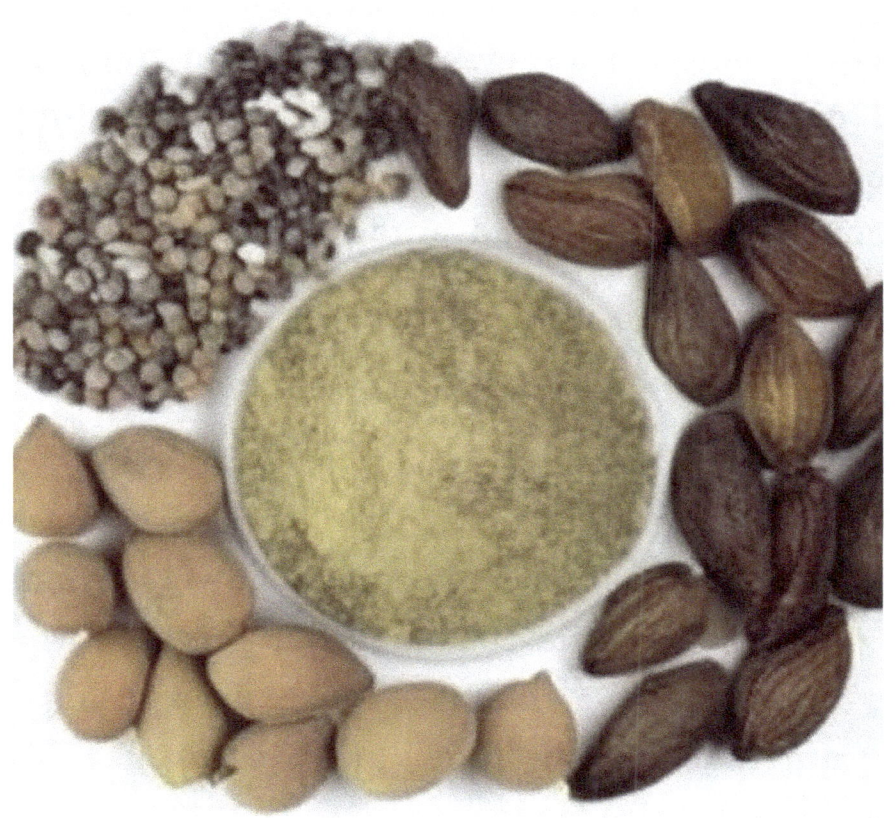

A combination of three fruits, aids digestion and detoxification.

Bibhitaki (Terminalia bellirica), Haritaki (Terminalia chebula), and Amalaki (Emblica officinalis) are the three fruits that make up the Ayurvedic herbal composition known as triphala. Many health advantages, especially in the areas of digestion and detoxification, are thought to come from this combination. The following are some possible health advantages of triphala:

1. Digestive health

- The benefits of Triphala for supporting and enhancing digestion are well known. It eases constipation and helps control bowel motions.
- The three fruits that make up triphala work together to enhance the absorption of nutrients from food and to arouse the digestive fire (agni).

2. Detoxification:
- Triphala is considered a mild laxative and helps in cleansing the gastrointestinal tract, aiding in the elimination of toxins from the body.

- It supports the liver's detoxification processes, promoting overall detoxification and purification of the body.

3. Properties of Antioxidants:

- Rich in antioxidants, the three fruits that make up Triphala aid in the body's defense against free radicals. This may help to lessen inflammation and oxidative stress.

4. Support for the Immune System:

- The high vitamin C concentration of triphala, especially from the Amalaki fruit, is thought to have immune-boosting effects. An immune system in good health requires vitamin C.

5. Controlling Weight:

- Triphala supports a healthy metabolism and digestive system, which may help with weight management. It aids in the body's removal of waste and extra water.

6. Oral Health:

    - Triphala is believed to promote oral health by preventing gum diseases, reducing plaque formation, and supporting overall oral hygiene.

7. Anti-Inflammatory Effects:

    - Triphala has anti-inflammatory properties that may help in reducing inflammation in the body, supporting joint health, and alleviating conditions related to inflammation.

8. Balancing Doshas:

    - In Ayurveda, Triphala is considered tridoshic, meaning it helps balance all three doshas – Vata, Pitta, and Kapha. This makes it suitable for individuals with different constitutional types.

Although triphala has been used traditionally for its health advantages, individual responses may differ. It is best to speak with a healthcare provider before adding any new supplements to your regimen, particularly if you are using medication or already have health issues.

Ghee

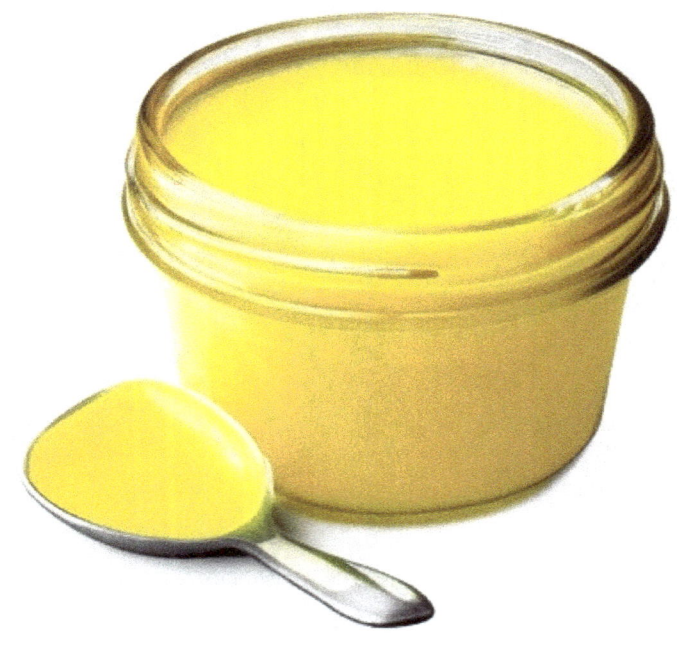

Clarified butter, supports digestion and immunity.

For ages, Indian traditional cookery has utilised ghee, which is a form of clarified butter. In order to make it, unsalted butter is simmered until the water evaporates and the milk solids separate from the golden liquid. Ghee is the name given to the leftover clarified butter.

Here are a few possible health advantages of ghee:

1. <u>**Rich in Good Fats:**</u> Although monounsaturated and polyunsaturated fats make up the majority of ghee's fat content, it also contains saturated fats. These fats can improve general well-being and are necessary for several body processes.

2. <u>**Lactose and Casein-Free:**</u> Ghee is acceptable for people who are intolerant to lactose or who are sensitive to dairy proteins because the clearing process eliminates the majority of the milk solids, including lactose and casein.

3. **High Smoke Point:** Ghee is a more stable frying fat than ordinary butter since it has a greater smoke point. This indicates that when used for cooking at high temperatures, it is less likely to decompose into dangerous free radicals.

4. **Rich in Fat-Soluble Vitamins:** Ghee contains fat-soluble vitamins such as A, D, E, and K. These vitamins play crucial roles in maintaining various bodily functions, including immune system support, bone health, and skin health.

5. **Supports Digestion:** Ghee is believed to stimulate the secretion of stomach acids, aiding in digestion. It is also thought to promote the health of the gut lining.

6. **May Boost Immunity:** Some studies suggest that ghee may have immune-boosting properties due to its content of butyric acid, which has been linked to improved immune function.

7. <u>Anti-Inflammatory Properties:</u> Ghee contains compounds like CLA (conjugated linoleic acid) and butyric acid, which may have anti-inflammatory effects. Chronic inflammation is associated with various health issues, so reducing inflammation can be beneficial.

8. <u>Ayurvedic Perspective:</u> In Ayurveda, the traditional system of medicine in India, ghee is considered to have numerous health benefits, including supporting overall well-being and vitality.

Moderation is vital when it comes to ghee because, despite its possible health benefits, it is still a high-calorie food. Personalised advice based on your unique health needs and situations can be obtained by consulting with a healthcare practitioner or nutritionist. Individual responses to dietary components can also differ.

Cardamom (Elaichi)

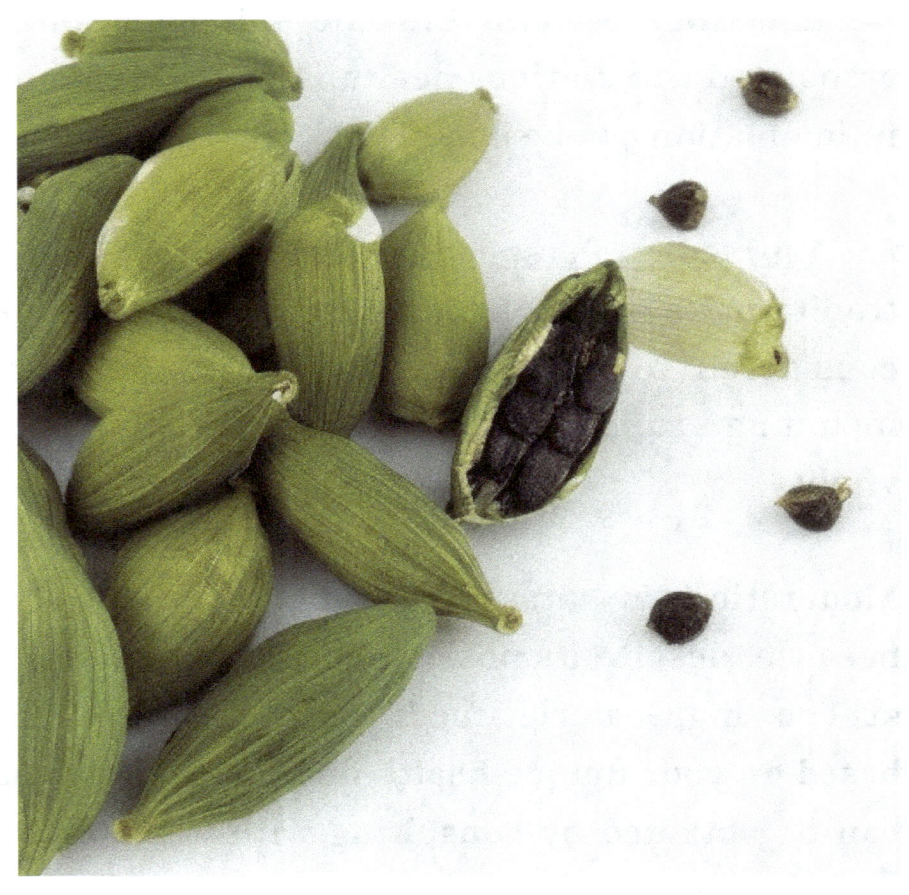

Improves digestion and freshens breath.

The word "Elaichi" alludes to cardamom, a spice derived from the seeds of various plants of the Zingiberaceae family's genera Elettaria and Amomum. Cardamom comes in two primary varieties: black cardamom (Amomum subulatum) and green cardamom (Elettaria cardamomum). Because of their unique flavours and scents, both varieties are utilised in a variety of cuisines.

The following are a few possible health advantages of cardamom:

1. Digestive Health: Cardamom is known to help with digestive issues such as indigestion, bloating, and gas. It may also stimulate the appetite and soothe an upset stomach.
2. Antioxidant Properties: Cardamom contains antioxidants that may help combat oxidative stress in the body, potentially reducing the risk of chronic diseases.
3. Anti-Inflammatory Effects: Some studies suggest that cardamom may have anti-inflammatory properties, which could be beneficial for conditions related to inflammation.

1. Heart Health: Cardamom may help lower blood pressure and improve overall heart health. It may also have a positive impact on cholesterol levels.
2. Oral Health: Traditionally, cardamom has been used to freshen breath and promote oral health. It is sometimes used in oral care products for its antimicrobial properties.
3. Respiratory Health: The aroma of cardamom may have a beneficial effect on respiratory health, helping to relieve symptoms of coughs and congestion.
4. Weight Management: Some studies suggest that cardamom may have potential benefits for weight management by improving metabolism and reducing appetite.

It's crucial to remember that although cardamom is a tasty spice with certain health advantages, these effects may differ from person to person and further study is required to determine the full scope of cardamom's impacts on health. Furthermore, it's a good idea to speak with a healthcare provider before making any big dietary or lifestyle changes, particularly if you already have any medical concerns.

Ajwain (Carom Seeds)

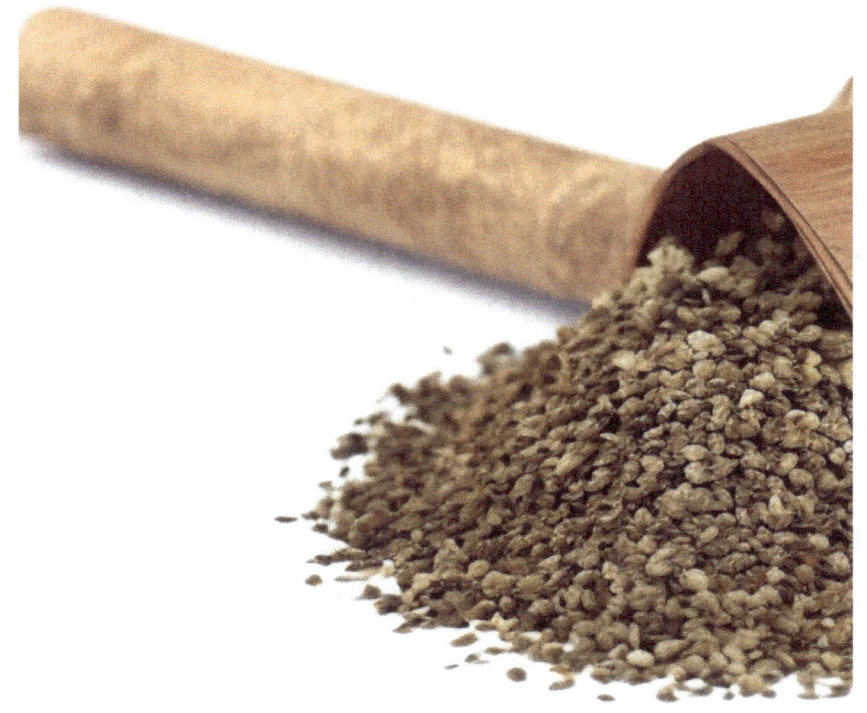

Relieves indigestion and gas.

In Indian cooking, ajwain, sometimes referred to as carom seeds, is a popular spice. It is made from the seeds of the Trachyspermum ammi, or ajwain plant. Ajwain is well-known for its unique flavour and scent, which are frequently characterised as strong and slightly bitter.

Ajwain is well renowned for its ability to reduce gas and indigestion, among other health advantages. The following are some possible health advantages of ajwain:

1. Digestive Aid: Ajwain contains active compounds like thymol, which can help in the secretion of digestive juices. It is believed to enhance the digestive process and alleviate indigestion, bloating, and gas.

2. Anti-inflammatory Properties: Ajwain is known for its anti-inflammatory properties, which may help in reducing inflammation in the digestive tract and other parts of the body.

3.Relief from Respiratory Issues: Ajwain is often used in traditional medicine to alleviate respiratory problems such as asthma, bronchitis, and congestion. The essential oil in Ajwain is believed to have bronchodilator and antimicrobial effects.

4.Antimicrobial Effects: The essential oil in Ajwain has been studied for its antimicrobial properties. It may have the ability to inhibit the growth of certain bacteria and fungi.

5.Anti-spasmodic Properties: Ajwain is considered to have anti-spasmodic effects, which means it may help in relaxing the muscles, providing relief from cramps and spasms.

6.Aids Weight Loss: Some people believe that Ajwain can aid in weight loss by boosting metabolism and promoting the burning of fat.

7.Rich in Nutrients: Ajwain contains various nutrients, including fiber, vitamins, and minerals, which contribute to overall health.

Although Ajwain has been traditionally utilised for its possible health advantages, individual responses may differ. Before adding new herbs or spices to your diet, it's a good idea to speak with a healthcare provider, particularly if you have any pre-existing health disorders or concerns.

Lemon (Nimbu)

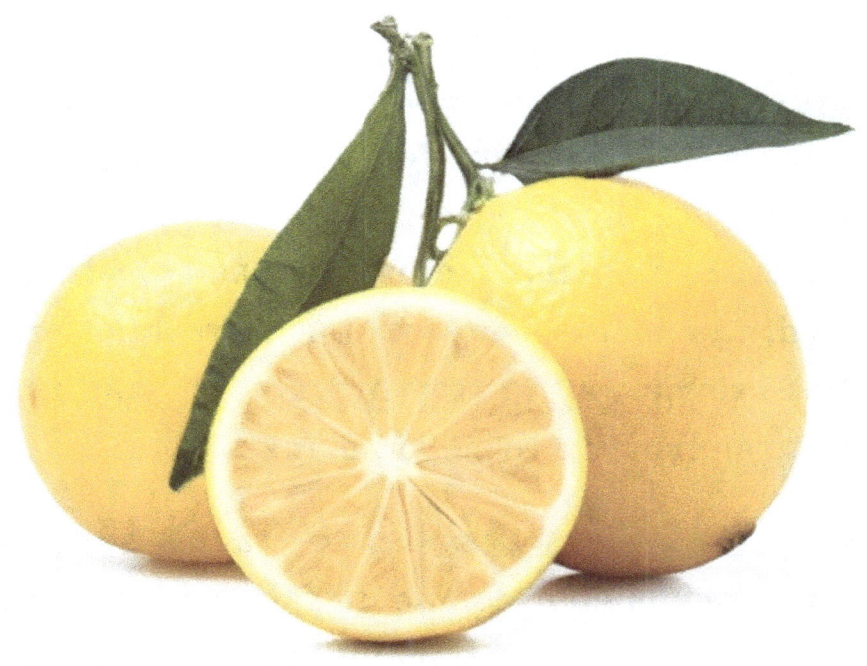

Detoxifies and provides Vitamin C.

Lemons are citrus fruits that are rich in various nutrients and have several health benefits. Here are some of the potential health benefits of lemons:

1. **High in Vitamin C**: Lemons are an excellent source of vitamin C, an antioxidant that helps boost the immune system, promotes skin health, and aids in the absorption of iron.
2. **Aids Digestion:** Lemon juice can help stimulate the production of digestive juices, promoting healthy digestion. It may also relieve symptoms of indigestion and bloating.
3. **Hydration**: Lemon water is a refreshing and low-calorie way to stay hydrated. It can be a good alternative to sugary drinks.

4. **Supports Weight Loss:** Some studies suggest that the polyphenol compounds in lemons may aid in weight loss. Additionally, the fiber content in lemons can help you feel full.

5. **Alkalizing Properties:** Despite being acidic in nature, lemons have an alkalizing effect on the body once metabolized. Maintaining a slightly alkaline pH may be beneficial for overall health.

6. <u>Skin Health</u>: The vitamin C in lemons plays a crucial role in collagen synthesis, contributing to healthy and vibrant skin. Lemon juice is also used topically for various skin-related issues.

7. <u>Rich in Potassium:</u> Lemons contain potassium, an essential mineral that helps regulate blood pressure, support heart health, and assist in proper muscle and nerve function.

8. <u>Antioxidant Properties</u>: The antioxidants in lemons, including vitamin C and flavonoids, help neutralize free radicals, which may contribute to aging and various diseases.

It's important to note that while lemons can be a healthy addition to your diet, consuming them in moderation is key, as excessive acidity may be harsh on tooth enamel. If you have specific health concerns or conditions, it's advisable to consult with a healthcare professional for personalized advice.

Sesame Oil (Til Tel)

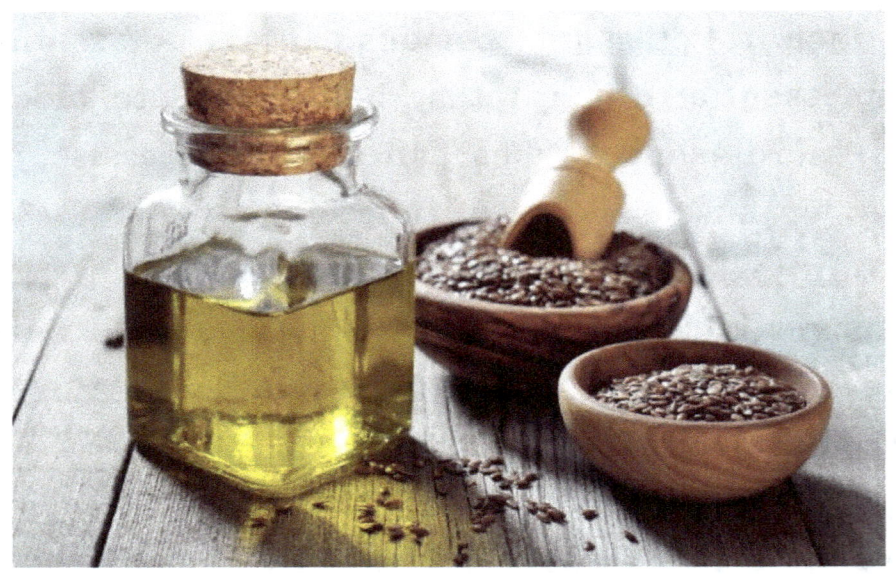

Used in oil pulling for oral health.

Vegetable oil made from sesame seeds is called sesame oil, or "Til Tel" in some places. It has been utilized in traditional medicine, skincare, and cuisine, among other things. Sesame oil is occasionally used in an oral hygiene procedure called "oil pulling." An old Ayurvedic practice known as "oil pulling" involves swishing oil about the mouth for a while to improve dental hygiene.

Here are some potential health benefits associated with sesame oil and its use in oil pulling for oral health:

1. Oral Health: Oil pulling with sesame oil is believed to help reduce harmful bacteria in the mouth, improve oral hygiene, and contribute to fresher breath. Some studies suggest that it may help in reducing plaque and gingivitis.
2. Antibacterial Properties: Sesame oil possesses antibacterial properties that may be beneficial for oral health. The oil may help inhibit the growth of bacteria in the mouth, reducing the risk of infections.

3. Anti-Inflammatory Effects: Sesame oil contains compounds with anti-inflammatory properties. This can be beneficial for reducing inflammation in the gums and promoting overall gum health.

4. Teeth Whitening: Some proponents of oil pulling claim that it can help whiten teeth by removing surface stains. However, more research is needed to support this claim.

5. Dry Mouth Relief: Sesame oil may help alleviate dry mouth symptoms. The oil's lubricating properties can help moisturize the mouth and reduce discomfort associated with dryness.

It's best to speak with a dentist or other healthcare provider before starting any new health regimen to make sure it meets your specific needs.

Castor Oil (Arandi Tel)

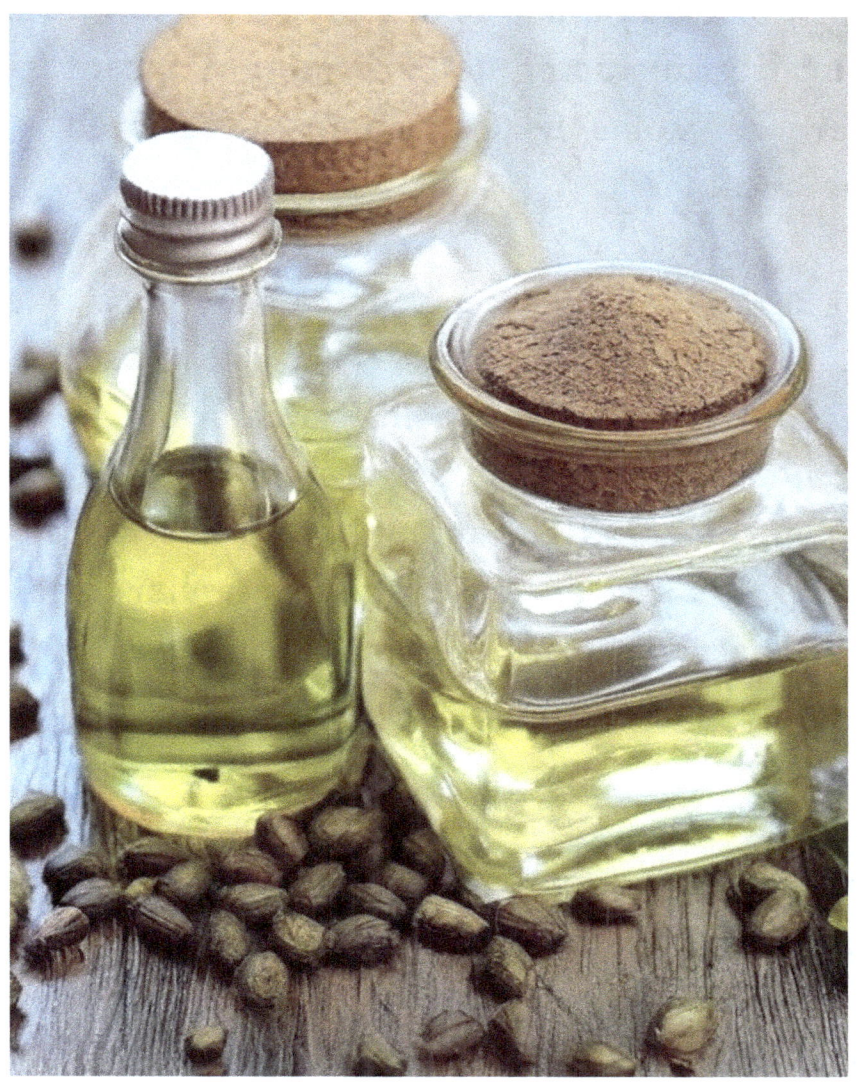

Used for various detoxification purposes.

Castor oil, also known as Arandi Tel in Hindi, is derived from the seeds of the castor plant (Ricinus communis). It has been used for various purposes, including detoxification, for centuries. Here are some health benefits associated with castor oil:

1. Laxative Properties: One of the most well-known uses of castor oil is as a laxative. It contains ricinoleic acid, which stimulates the muscles in the intestines, promoting bowel movements. It is important to use castor oil as a laxative cautiously and under medical supervision, as excessive use can lead to dehydration and electrolyte imbalance.

2. Skin Health: Castor oil has moisturizing properties, making it beneficial for the skin. It is often used in skincare products to alleviate dry skin and conditions like eczema. Some people also use it for acne, although individual responses may vary.

3. **Anti-Inflammatory Effects:** The ricinoleic acid in castor oil has anti-inflammatory properties. This makes it useful for reducing inflammation and relieving pain associated with conditions such as arthritis or sore muscles.

4. **Detoxification:** Castor oil has been traditionally used for detoxification purposes. It is believed to help the body eliminate toxins by promoting bowel movements. Some alternative medicine practitioners recommend castor oil packs applied to the abdomen to support detoxification processes.

5. **Hair Care:** Castor oil is often used in hair care for its moisturizing properties. It can help nourish the hair and scalp, potentially promoting hair growth and reducing dandruff.

6. **Immune System Support:** Some studies suggest that ricinoleic acid, found in castor oil, may have immune-boosting properties. However, more research is needed to fully understand its impact on the immune system.

7. Anti-Fungal Properties: Castor oil may be useful in treating fungal infections of the skin or nails due to its potential anti-fungal qualities.

It's crucial to remember that even while castor oil has several potential advantages, using it should be done so carefully. Adverse reactions may result from misuse or overuse. It is best to speak with a healthcare provider before taking castor oil for any health-related purpose to be sure it is safe and suitable for your particular circumstance.

Trikatu Churna

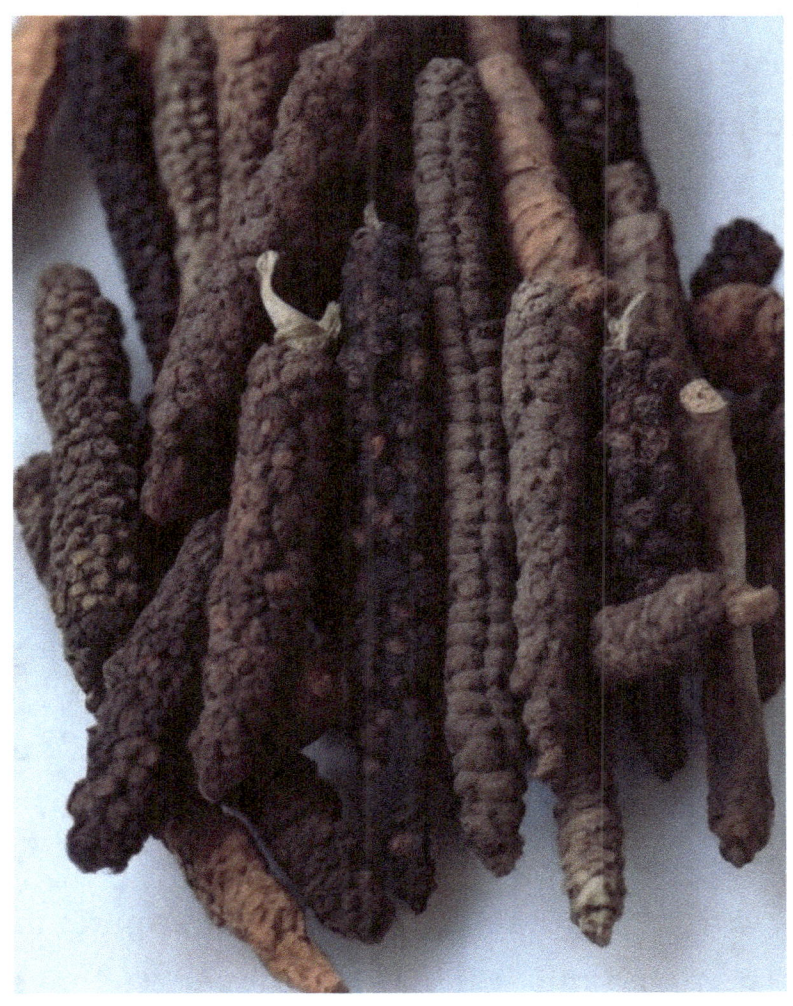

A blend of black pepper, long pepper, and ginger for digestion.

Three essential ingredients make up the traditional Ayurvedic herbal formula known as Trikatu Churna: ginger (Zingiber officinale), long pepper (Piper longum), and black pepper (Piper nigrum). Trikatu Churna, renowned for its medicinal and digestive qualities, is made using a precise ratio of these three spices. The following are some possible health advantages of trikatu churna:

1. Digestive Aid:
   - Trikatu Churna is primarily known for its digestive properties. It stimulates the digestive fire (agni) in the body, promoting efficient digestion and absorption of nutrients.
   - It may help alleviate digestive issues such as indigestion, bloating, and flatulence.
2. Metabolism Boost:
   - The combination of black pepper, long pepper, and ginger is believed to have a thermogenic effect, potentially boosting metabolism and promoting weight management.

3. Respiratory Health:

Ginger and black pepper have traditionally been used to support respiratory health. Trikatu Churna may help in managing respiratory conditions such as cough and congestion.

4. Circulation Improvement:

Black pepper is known for its potential to improve blood circulation. This can contribute to overall cardiovascular health.

5. Anti-Inflammatory Properties:

The individual components of Trikatu, particularly ginger, possess anti-inflammatory properties that may help in reducing inflammation in the body.

6. Detoxification:

Trikatu Churna is believed to have detoxifying effects, helping the body eliminate waste and toxins.

7. point Health:
   - The anti-inflammatory properties of Trikatu may also be beneficial for joint health, potentially providing relief from conditions like arthritis.

8. Immune Support:
   - Some of the ingredients, especially ginger, are known for their immune-boosting properties, contributing to overall wellness.

9. Enhanced Nutrient Absorption:
   - By promoting healthy digestion, Trikatu Churna may enhance the absorption of nutrients from the food we consume.

Although Trikatu Churna has been used for a very long time in traditional Ayurvedic therapy, it's vital to remember that different people react differently to herbal supplements. Speak with a healthcare provider before adding any new supplements to your regimen, particularly if you have any underlying medical concerns or are currently taking other prescriptions.

BRAMHI

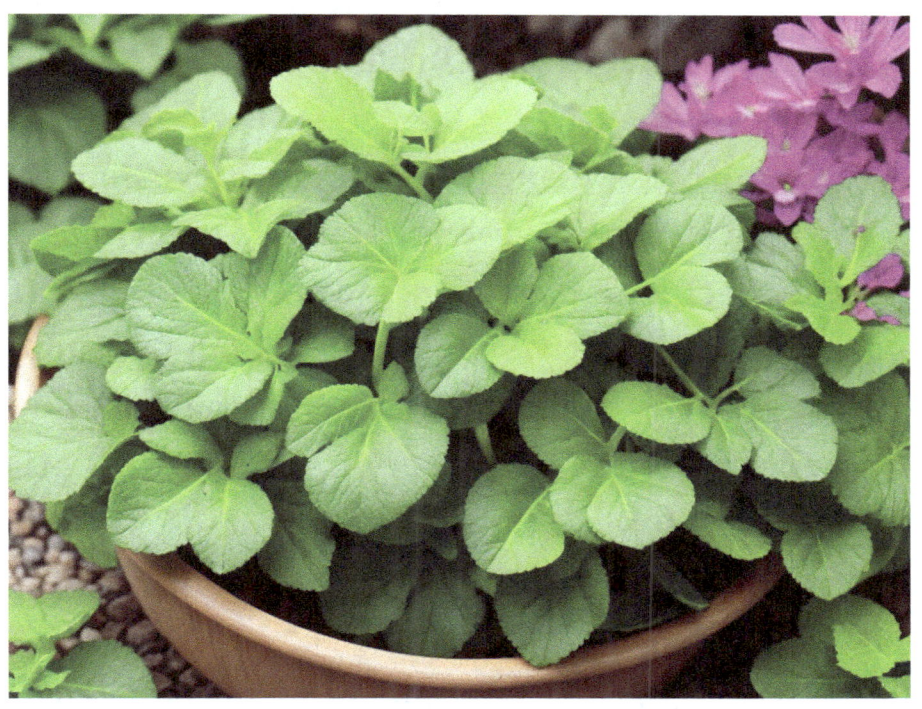

Improves cognitive function and reduces stress.

Brahmi, scientifically known as Bacopa monnieri, is a herb that has been used in traditional Ayurvedic medicine for centuries. It is known for its potential health benefits, particularly in improving cognitive function and reducing stress. Here are some of the potential health benefits associated with Brahmi:

1. <u>Cognitive Enhancement:</u> Brahmi is believed to have cognitive-enhancing properties. It may help improve memory, learning, and overall cognitive function. Some studies suggest that Brahmi may have neuroprotective effects, promoting the growth of nerve cells and enhancing synaptic transmission.

2. <u>Stress Reduction</u>: Brahmi is often considered an adaptogen, which means it may help the body adapt to stress and maintain balance. It is thought to have anxiolytic (anxiety-reducing) properties, potentially helping to alleviate stress and anxiety.

3. <u>Anti-Inflammatory Properties</u>: The potential anti-inflammatory benefits of Brahmi have been investigated. Brahmi's anti-inflammatory qualities may improve general well-being because chronic inflammation is linked to a number of health problems.

4. <u>Antioxidant Activity</u>: The antioxidant-rich chemicals found in Brahmi can aid in the body's defense against damaging free radicals. Antioxidants may improve general health as well as shield cells from oxidative damage.

5. <u>Enhanced Mood</u>: According to certain studies, Brahmi may improve mood and lessen the signs and symptoms of depression. To completely understand its impact on mood disorders, more research is necessary.

6. <u>Improved Sleep</u>: Brahmi has the capacity to soothe the nervous system and improve the quality of sleep. Having more quality sleep can benefit one's general health and wellbeing.

7. **Anti-Anxiety Effects**: Brahmi's anxiolytic qualities may aid in lowering anxiety symptoms. It's thought to affect specific neurotransmitters in the brain, which helps to calm things down.

It is noteworthy that although Brahmi has potential in multiple health domains, further investigation is imperative to comprehensively comprehend its mechanisms and their enduring consequences. Furthermore, because Brahmi can have different effects on different people, it's best to speak with a healthcare provider before using it regularly, particularly if you have any underlying medical conditions or are on medication.

Shatavari

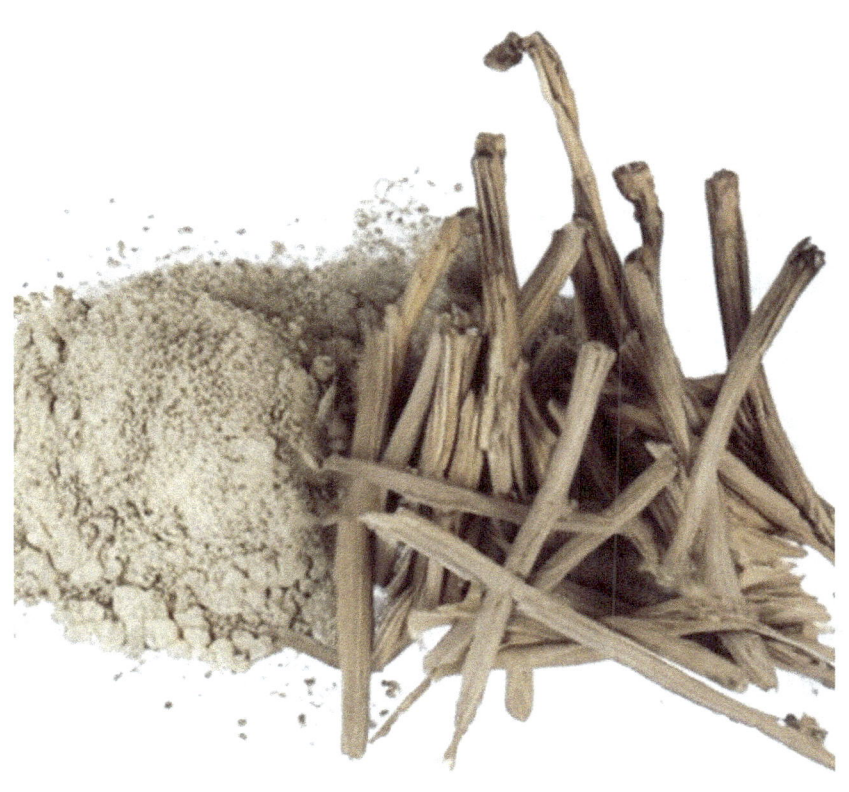

Supports female reproductive health.

Traditionally used for millennia in Ayurvedic medicine, Shatavari, formally known as Asparagus racemosus, is a herb with potential benefits for maintaining female reproductive health. The following are a few possible health advantages of Shatavari:

1. <u>Menstrual Health</u>: It is thought that shatavari balances the female reproductive system and may aid in menstrual cycle regulation. It is frequently used to reduce menstruation-related symptoms like cramping and mood swings.

2. <u>Fertility Support</u>: Shatavari has been traditionally used for its potential to support women's fertility. It is thought to support general reproductive health and nourish the female reproductive organs.

3. <u>Menopausal Support:</u> Shatavari may help ease symptoms associated with menopause, such as hot flashes, mood swings, and irritability. Its phytoestrogenic properties are thought to contribute to hormonal balance.

4. Shatavari is regarded as a uterine tonic, which implies that it could aid in toning and fortifying the uterus. This may promote a healthy pregnancy and be advantageous for reproductive health in general.

5. immunological System Support: Shatavari may be able to strengthen the body's immunological response because of its immunomodulatory qualities.

6. Anti-Inflammatory Properties: The herb may contain anti-inflammatory properties that make it useful for conditions where the reproductive system is inflamed.

7. Adaptogenic Properties: Shatavari is categorized as an adaptogen, meaning it has the potential to assist the body in balancing and adapting to stress. The general well-being, which includes reproductive health, may benefit from this.

While shatavari has a long history of usage in traditional medicine and is generally regarded as safe, it's crucial to remember that individual responses may differ. It is best to speak with a healthcare provider before using Shatavari or any other herbal supplement, particularly if you are expecting, nursing, or using other medications. Furthermore, Shatavari is still being studied scientifically, and more data is required to completely comprehend the benefits and modes of action of this herb.

Guduchi (Giloy)

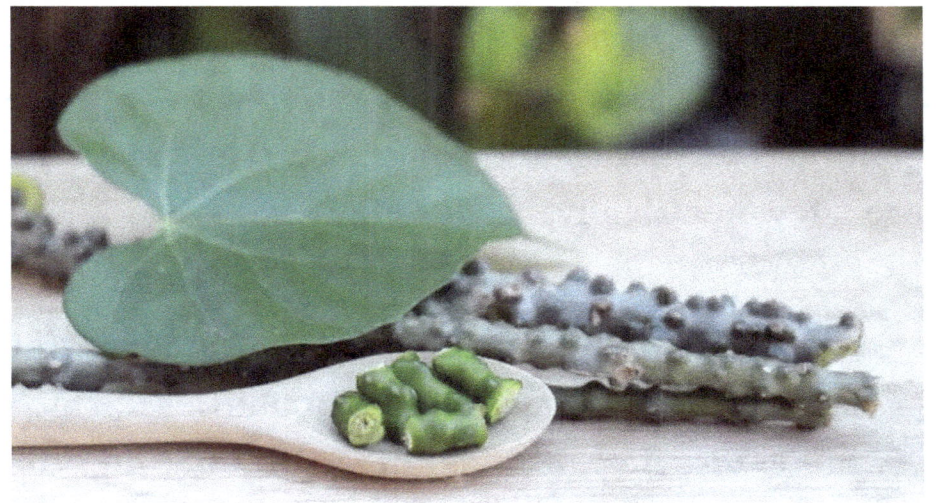

Boosts immunity and aids in fever.

For millennia, Ayurvedic medicine has utilised giloy, also called Tinospora cordifolia, as a medicinal herb. It is sometimes called "Amrita" in Sanskrit, which translates as "root of immortality." Giloy is well-known for its many health advantages and is regarded in Ayurveda as a Rasayana, which means it is thought to enhance general well-being and longevity. The following are a few health advantages of giloy:

1. **Boosts Immunity:** Giloy is well known for having immunomodulatory qualities, which indicates that it aids in strengthening the immunological system of the body. It might aid the body's defence against illnesses and infections.

2. **Anti-inflammatory:** Giloy has anti-inflammatory qualities that could aid in the body's reduction of swelling and inflammation. In cases of arthritis and other inflammatory illnesses, this may be helpful.

3. <u>Antioxidant Properties:</u> The herb is rich in antioxidants, which can help neutralize free radicals in the body. This may contribute to preventing oxidative stress and reducing the risk of chronic diseases.

4. <u>Fever Reduction</u>: Giloy is known for its antipyretic properties, making it useful in managing fever. It is often used in Ayurvedic formulations to treat various types of fevers.

5. <u>Detoxification</u>: It is believed that Giloy can help in detoxifying the body by removing toxins and purifying the blood. This can contribute to overall health and well-being.

6. <u>Diabetes Management</u>: Some studies suggest that Giloy may have hypoglycemic effects, helping in managing blood sugar levels. However, more research is needed in this area.

7. <u>Respiratory Health:</u> Giloy is used traditionally to treat respiratory problems such as asthma, bronchitis, and cough. It is believed to have mucolytic properties, aiding in the removal of mucus from the respiratory tract.

8. <u>Digestive Health</u>: The herb may be used to treat a variety of digestive issues and to improve digestion. It is said to have carminative qualities, which lessen pain and flatulence.

9. <u>Adaptogenic Properties</u>: Because Giloy is an adaptogen, it may aid the body in balancing and adapting to stress. On the whole, this may be beneficial to health.

Though Giloy has many potential health benefits, individual responses may differ. As such, it is best to speak with a healthcare provider before introducing Giloy into your routine, particularly if you have any underlying medical conditions or are currently taking other medications. Furthermore, further research is required to completely comprehend the degree of Giloy's medicinal benefits because the information presented here is based on traditional applications and a few scientific investigations.

Mulethi (Licorice)

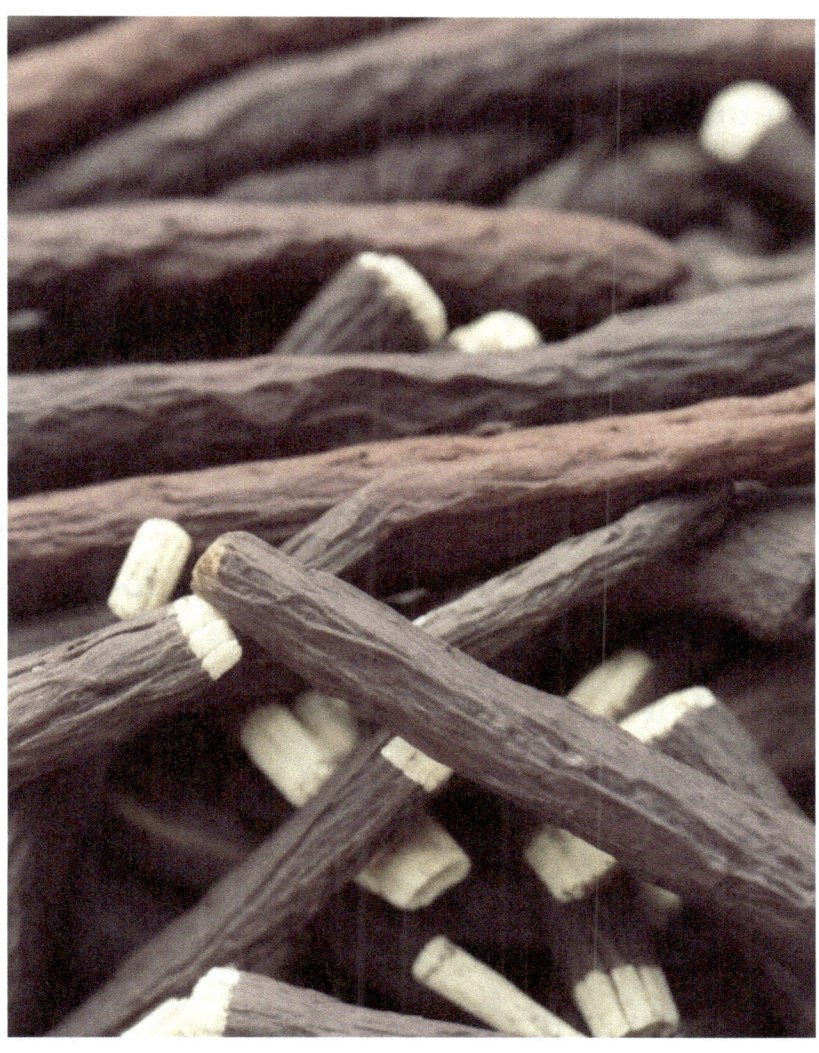

Soothes sore throat and supports respiratory health.

Mulethi, botanically known as Glycyrrhiza glabra or Licorice, is a herb that has been utilised for ages in traditional medicine, particularly in Ayurveda. It is indigenous to some regions of Asia and the Mediterranean. Due to its many health advantages, licorice root is frequently used. The following are some possible health advantages of mulethi:

- <u>Anti-Inflammatory Properties</u>: Glycyrrhizin, a substance found in mulethi, has anti-inflammatory qualities. It might aid in the body's reduction of inflammation.

- <u>Cough and Respiratory Health</u>: Licorice is frequently used to treat respiratory conditions like sore throats and coughs. It is thought to contain expectorant qualities, which aid in clearing the respiratory tract of mucus.

- **Digestive Health**: Mulethi is known to have mild laxative effects and may help in maintaining a healthy digestive system. It is used to treat issues like indigestion, heartburn, and acidity.

- **Anti-viral and Anti-bacterial**: Some studies suggest that licorice may have antiviral and antibacterial properties, making it potentially beneficial for combating infections.

- **Skin Benefits**: Mulethi is believed to have skin-soothing properties. It is used in various skincare products to help with issues like eczema and dermatitis.

- **Hormonal Balance**: Licorice may influence hormonal balance by affecting cortisol levels. It has been traditionally used in women's health to alleviate symptoms related to hormonal imbalances.

- Adrenal Support: Research indicates that licorice may assist the adrenal glands in their work, which in turn helps the body handle stress.

- Effects against diabetes: Some studies suggest that licorice may help people with diabetes manage their blood sugar levels.

Notwithstanding these possible advantages, it's crucial to remember that consuming too much licorice, especially glycyrrhizin, might have negative effects like elevated blood pressure, potassium loss, and other illnesses. It is advised to use licorice sparingly and to speak with a doctor, particularly if you are on medication or have pre-existing medical conditions.

Haritaki

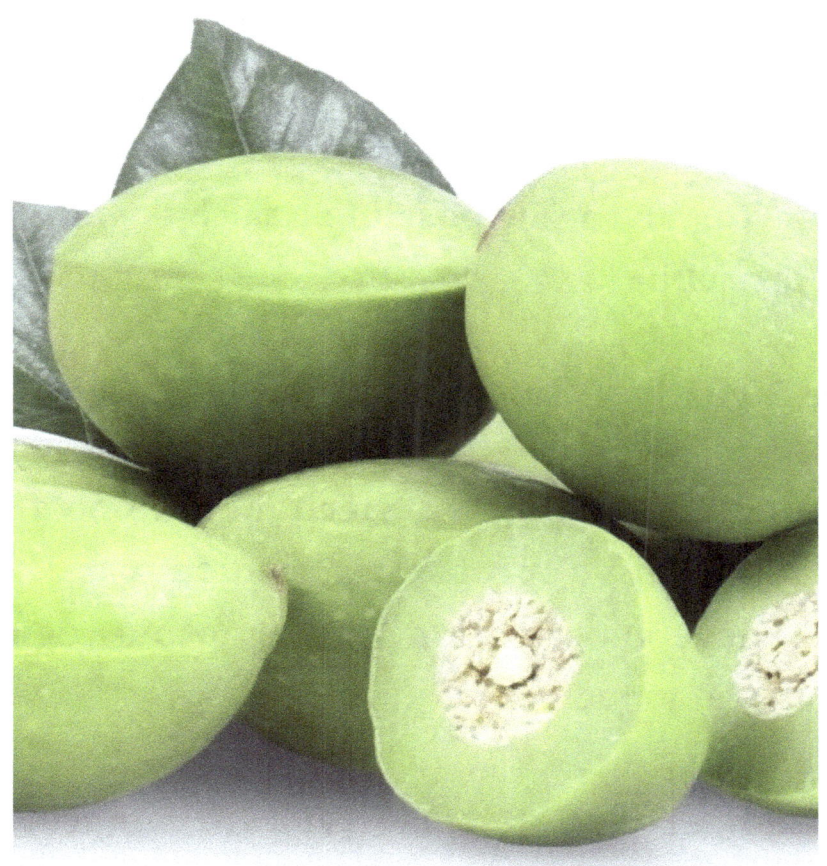

Promotes digestive health and detoxification.

The fruit haritaki, also called Terminalia chebula, has been utilised for millennia in traditional Ayurvedic medicine, an Indian system of natural treatment. It is thought that haritaki has a number of health advantages, especially in terms of supporting detoxification and digestive health. The following are a few possible health advantages of Haritaki:

1. Digestive Health:

- **Constipation Relief:** Haritaki is known for its laxative properties, which can help relieve constipation by promoting regular bowel movements.

- **Indigestion:** It may aid in improving digestion and reducing symptoms of indigestion by enhancing the digestive process.

2. Detoxification:
    - **Colon Cleansing: Haritaki is believed to help cleanse the colon, removing toxins and promoting a healthier digestive tract.**
    - **Liver Health: It may support liver function and help in detoxifying the body by eliminating harmful substances.**

3. Antioxidant Properties:
    - **Haritaki contains antioxidants that can help neutralize free radicals in the body, potentially protecting cells from damage.**

4. Anti-inflammatory Effects:
    - **Some studies suggest that Haritaki may have anti-inflammatory properties, which could be beneficial in managing inflammatory conditions.**

5. Weight Management:
   - Haritaki may be helpful in weight management by promoting healthy digestion and metabolism.

6. Respiratory Health:
   - In traditional medicine, Haritaki is also used to address respiratory issues and promote lung health.

7. Improves Oral Health:
   - Haritaki is believed to have antimicrobial properties that can help maintain oral hygiene and prevent dental issues.

8. Supports Immune System:
   - The antioxidants present in Haritaki may contribute to supporting the immune system by reducing oxidative stress.

It's important to note that while Haritaki has a long history of use in traditional medicine, scientific research on its specific health benefits is still ongoing. Before incorporating Haritaki or any herbal supplement into your routine, it's advisable to consult with a healthcare professional, especially if you have pre-existing medical conditions or are taking other medications. Individual responses to herbal remedies can vary, and caution should be exercised to ensure safety and effectiveness.

Bhringraj Oil

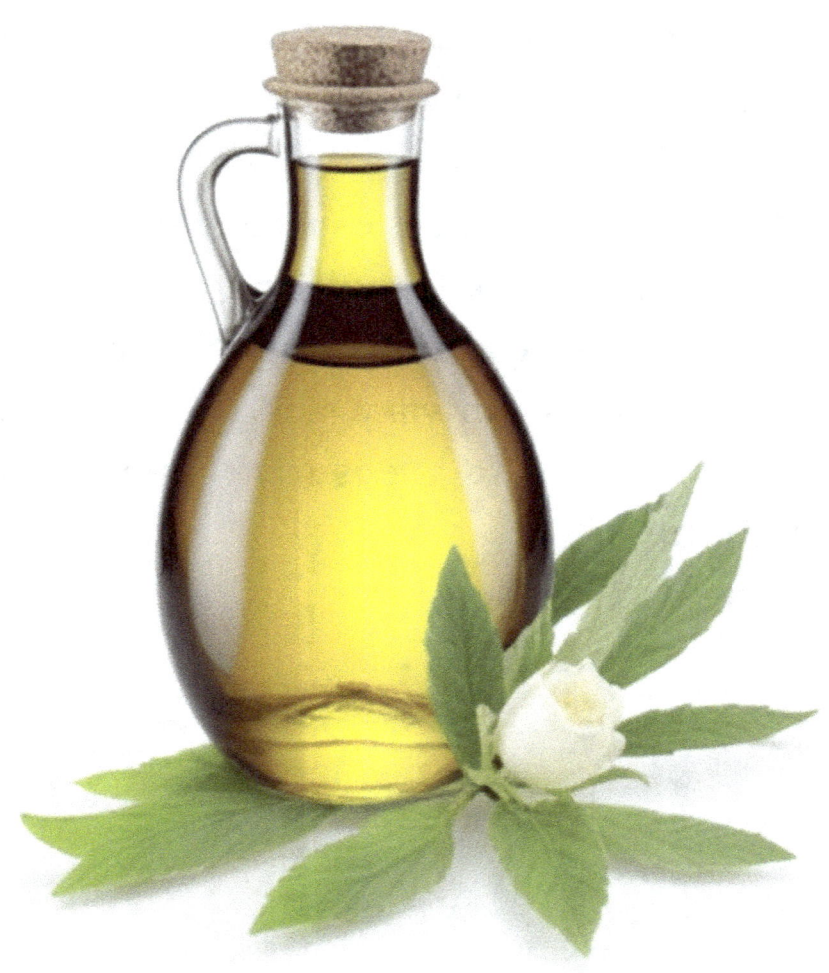

Nourishes hair and promotes hair growth.

The scientific name for the Bhringraj plant, Eclipta alba, is where "Bhringraj oil" is from. Because of this plant's many health and hair care advantages, Ayurvedic medicine has long employed it. Particularly well-liked for its possible benefits to the health of the hair and scalp is Bhringraj oil. These are a few of its cited advantages:

1. Hair Growth: Bhringraj oil is frequently used to stop hair loss and encourage hair growth. It is thought to increase blood flow to the scalp and activate hair follicles, promoting the development of robust, healthy hair.

2. Preventing Premature Greying: It is believed that using Bhringraj oil regularly can help stop hair from greying too soon. It is thought to support hair follicles and stop the fading of natural hair colour.

1. <u>Dandruff Control:</u> Bhringraj oil is considered effective in controlling dandruff and other scalp conditions. It has antimicrobial properties that may help in maintaining a healthy scalp.
2. <u>Conditioning:</u> The oil is often used as a natural conditioner. It helps in making the hair soft, smooth, and manageable by providing essential nutrients to the hair shaft.
3. <u>Reducing Split Ends</u>: Bhringraj oil may help in reducing split ends and preventing breakage. It nourishes the hair and strengthens it from root to tip.
4. <u>Scalp Health</u>: Bhringraj oil is known to have anti-inflammatory properties that can help in maintaining a healthy scalp. It may soothe irritated scalp conditions and reduce inflammation.
5. <u>Cooling Effect</u>: In Ayurveda, Bhringraj is considered to have a cooling effect, which can be beneficial for calming the scalp and reducing heat-related issues.

Although Bhringraj oil has been traditionally used for these purposes, there is a paucity of scientific data on its efficacy, and individual experiences may differ. Do a patch test before using any new supplement or hair care product to make sure there are no negative effects. If you have any specific concerns, speak with a healthcare provider or a hair care expert.

Gotu Kola (Mandukaparni)

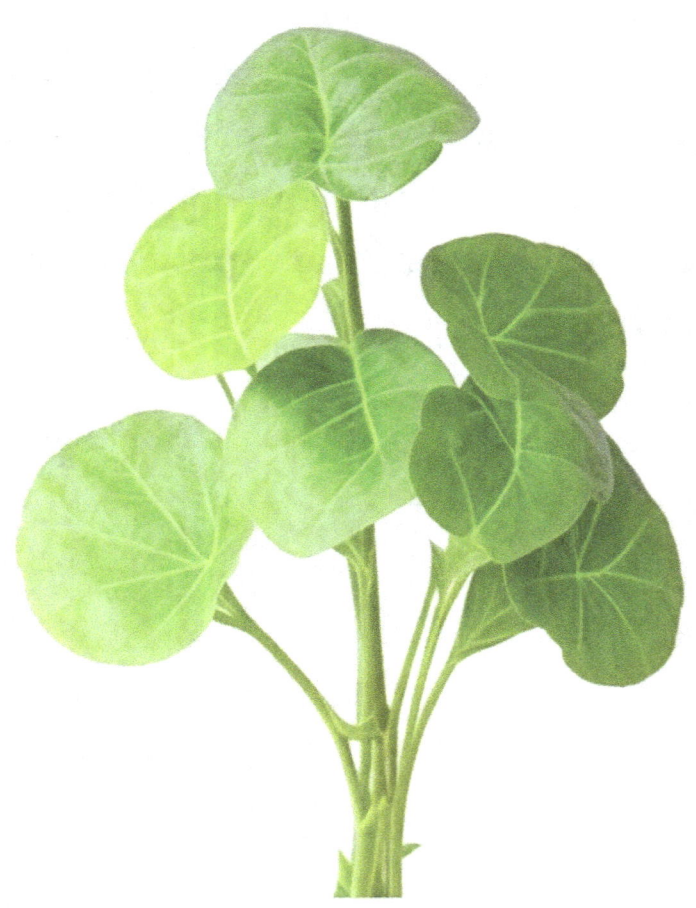

Supports cognitive function and skin health.

The herbaceous plant gotu kola, also called Mandukaparni or Centella asiatica, has long been utilised in many traditional medical systems, especially in Asian civilizations like Ayurveda and traditional Chinese medicine. It is well-known for its possible health advantages, which include promoting skin and cognitive performance. Here are a few possible advantages:

1. Cognitive Function:

- Memory Enhancement: Gotu Kola is believed to have cognitive-enhancing properties, and it is often used to support memory and concentration.
- Brain Health: Some studies suggest that Gotu Kola may have neuroprotective effects, which could contribute to overall brain health.

2. Skin Health:
   - **Collagen Production:** Gotu Kola is thought to stimulate the production of collagen, a protein important for maintaining skin elasticity and promoting wound healing.
   - **Wound Healing:** The herb has been used traditionally for wound healing and is believed to have properties that support tissue regeneration.

3. Antioxidant Properties:
   - Gotu Kola contains compounds with antioxidant properties, which may help protect cells from oxidative stress and reduce inflammation.

4. Anti-Anxiety and Antidepressant Effects:
   - Some research suggests that Gotu Kola may have mild anxiolytic (anxiety-reducing) and antidepressant effects, potentially contributing to overall mental well-being.

5. The insufficiency of veins :
- **Gotu Kola has been used to treat venous insufficiency, a disorder in which the walls of the veins weaken and cause blood to pool in the legs. It might aid in enhancing circulation and lowering pain and swelling symptoms.**

6. Effects against Inflammation:
- **The herb may help with inflammatory problems because it is thought to have anti-inflammatory effects.**

It is noteworthy that although Gotu Kola has been traditionally used for a long time and has been supported by some scientific studies for its potential advantages, further research is necessary to completely understand its mechanisms and determine its efficacy for different health issues. Furthermore, each person may react differently to herbal supplements, so it's best to speak with a healthcare provider before starting a supplement regimen, particularly if you have a medical history or are already taking medication.

Aloe Vera

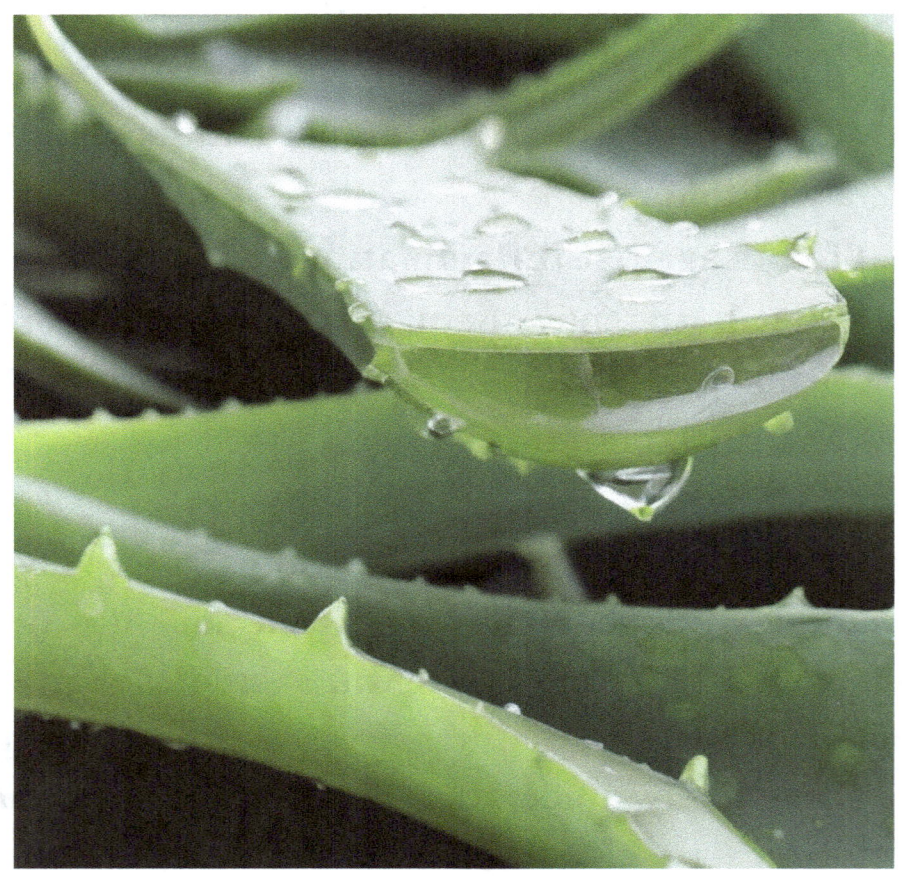

Supports skin health and digestion.

The succulent plant species aloe vera is well known for its many health advantages. The following are some of the main advantages of aloe vera:

1. <u>Skin Health</u>: The advantages of aloe vera for skin health are arguably the most well-known. It has ingredients with wound-healing, antibacterial, and anti-inflammatory qualities. It helps relieve ailments including sunburn, small burns, wounds, and abrasions by soothing and moisturizing the skin. Aloe vera gel is frequently found in skincare products like gels, lotions, and creams.
2. Digestive Health: Due to its possible advantages for digestive health, aloe vera juice is frequently ingested. It has ingredients like polysaccharides, which may calm the gastrointestinal system. Aloe vera juice is used by some people to assist relieve the symptoms of gastrointestinal disorders like acid reflux, constipation, and irritable bowel syndrome (IBS). However, it's important to use aloe vera juice sparingly because taking too much of it can cause upset stomach or other negative effects.

3. Immune Support: Aloe vera contains various vitamins, minerals, and antioxidants that can help support the immune system. These nutrients may help the body defend against pathogens and reduce inflammation, potentially contributing to overall immune health.

4. Hydration: Aloe vera gel is rich in water content and can help hydrate the skin when applied topically. Additionally, drinking aloe vera juice can contribute to hydration, as it provides water along with various nutrients.

5. Nutrient-Rich: Aloe vera contains vitamins (such as vitamins A, C, and E), minerals (such as calcium, magnesium, and zinc), enzymes, amino acids, and other beneficial compounds. These nutrients play various roles in supporting overall health and well-being.

6. Antioxidant Properties: Aloe vera contains antioxidants that help combat oxidative stress and damage caused by free radicals in the body. Regular consumption or topical application of aloe vera may help protect cells from damage and reduce the risk of chronic diseases associated with oxidative stress.

7. Oral Health: Aloe vera may enhance oral health, according to certain research. When used to mouthwash or toothpaste, it may help lessen oral infections, gum irritation, and plaque accumulation. Further investigation is need to completely validate these possible advantages, though.

It's crucial to remember that although aloe vera may have a number of health benefits, each person may react differently, and some may have allergic reactions or other negative side effects. Before utilizing aloe vera supplements or applying aloe vera products, it's always a good idea to speak with a healthcare provider, particularly if you have any underlying medical concerns or are taking medication.

Arjuna

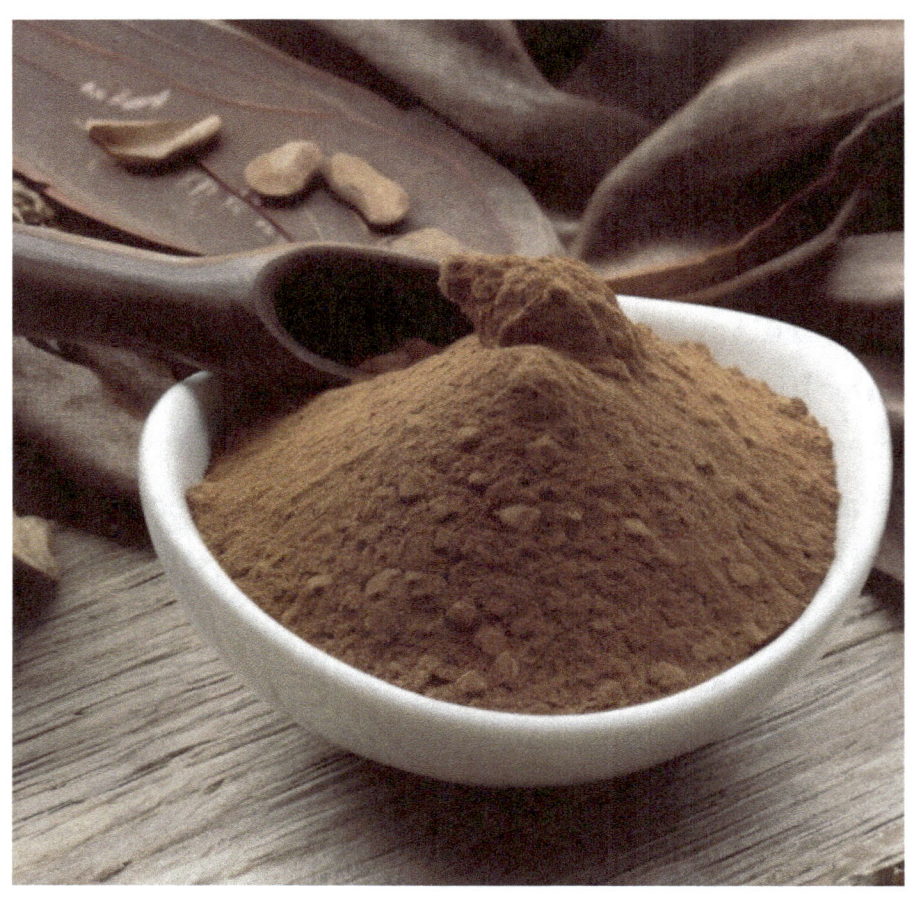

ASupports cardiovascular health.

The bark of the native Indian Terminalia arjuna tree is used to make the therapeutic herb arjuna. It has been used for ages to promote cardiovascular health in traditional Ayurvedic treatment. Some of its health advantages are as follows:

1. Heart Health: The main advantage of arjuna is said to be for the cardiovascular system. Flavonoids, tannins, and minerals are among the components it contains that support improved circulation, blood pressure regulation, and heart muscle strength. It is thought to possess cardioprotective qualities, which could aid in the treatment of ailments including angina and hypertension.

2. Reduces Cholesterol: Studies on the lipid-reducing effects of arjuna have shown that it can raise HDL cholesterol, the "good" cholesterol, while lowering total cholesterol and LDL cholesterol, the "bad" cholesterol. This can lower the risk of heart disease and help to create a healthy lipid profile.

3. **Anti-inflammatory Effects:** Arjuna contains compounds with anti-inflammatory properties, which may help reduce inflammation in the cardiovascular system. Chronic inflammation is associated with various heart conditions, so reducing inflammation can be beneficial for overall heart health.

4. **Antioxidant Activity:** The herb is rich in antioxidants, including flavonoids and polyphenols, which help neutralize harmful free radicals in the body. By reducing oxidative stress, arjuna may protect the heart and blood vessels from damage caused by free radicals, thus lowering the risk of cardiovascular diseases.

5. **Improves Heart Function:** Arjuna is known to improve the contractility of the heart muscles, which means it helps the heart pump blood more efficiently. This can lead to better overall heart function and may benefit individuals with conditions like heart failure or weakened heart muscles.

6. **Stress Management:** Arjuna may have adaptogenic qualities, which means it aids the body in adjusting to stress and preserving equilibrium, according to some research. Reducing stress can help cardiovascular health indirectly because stress can have detrimental consequences on the heart.

7. **Boosts Exercise Performance:** Research has indicated that arjuna may increase endurance and tolerance to exercise. It might facilitate better blood flow and cardiovascular support, which would enable people to participate in physical activity more successfully—a vital component of good health overall.

It is noteworthy that although arjuna has potential in enhancing cardiovascular well-being, further investigation is necessary to comprehensively comprehend its modes of action and its efficacy across all demographics.

Trikatu Churna

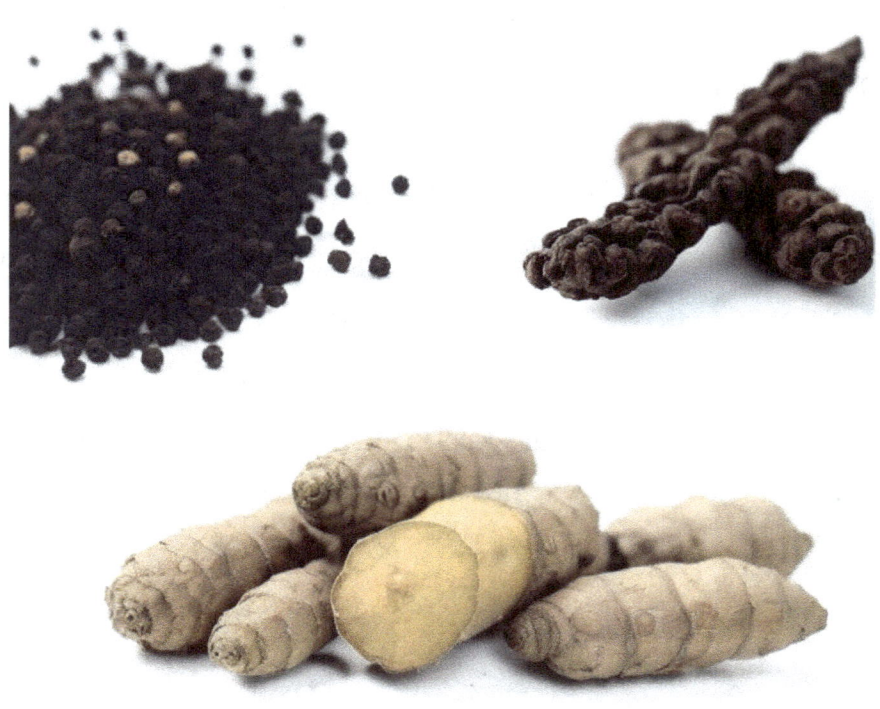

A blend of ginger, black pepper, and long pepper for digestion.

Three essential ingredients make up the ancient Ayurvedic herbal combination known as trikatu churna: ginger (Zingiber officinale), long pepper (Piper longum), and black pepper (Piper nigrum). In Ayurveda, this combination is well known for its many health advantages, especially for improving digestion. The following are a few possible health advantages of trikatu churna:

1. Digestive Aid: The main purpose of a triptu churna is to improve digestion. Digestive aids include ginger, long pepper, and black pepper. They enhance appetite, encourage good digestion, and increase the secretion of digestive juices—all of which can help reduce symptoms such as indigestion, gas, and bloating.

2. Metabolism Booster: It is thought that the chemicals in Trikatu Churna have thermogenic qualities, which means they can aid in raising metabolic rate. This may help with fat metabolism and weight control.

3. **Respiratory Health:** Expectorants, such as ginger, black pepper, and long pepper, can help treat respiratory ailments such congestion, coughing, and colds. Additionally, they might facilitate better breathing and respiratory passage clearance.

4. **Anti-inflammatory Effects:** Trikatu churna's components have anti-inflammatory qualities that may aid in lowering the body's level of inflammation. For ailments including inflammatory bowel illnesses and arthritis, this might be helpful.

5. **Improved Circulation:** It is well known that long and black peppers help to increase blood flow. This may help transport nutrients to different areas of the body and have a good impact on cardiovascular health in general.

6. **Detoxification:** It is said that trikatu churna aids in the body's detoxification procedures, assisting in the removal of waste materials and poisons. This may enhance overall

7. Immune Support: The chemicals in ginger, black pepper, and long pepper may help strengthen the immune system, increasing the body's resistance to diseases and infections.

8. Enhancement of Appetite: Trikatu churna is good for people who have trouble digesting food or who don't eat much because it can increase appetite.

Though Trikatu churna has been used for centuries in traditional Ayurvedic medicine and is generally regarded as safe, it is best to speak with a healthcare provider before starting any new herbal remedy regimen, particularly if you are taking medication or have pre-existing health conditions.

Dandelion Tea

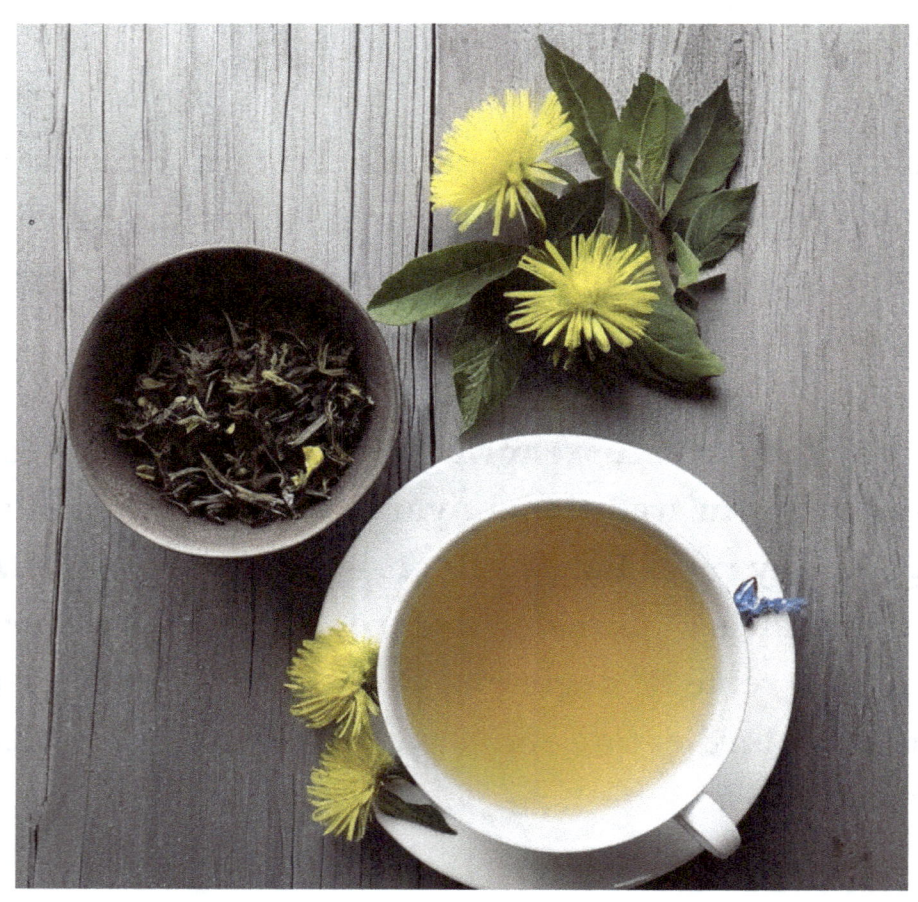

Supports liver health and digestion.

Scientifically called as Taraxacum officinale, dandelion tea is an infusion of herbs prepared from the leaves, petals, or roots of the dandelion plant. Its possible health benefits have led to its traditional use in many cultures. The following are some alleged advantages of dandelion tea:

1. Liver Health: Dandelion tea is often touted for its liver-cleansing properties. It may help support liver function by stimulating the flow of bile, which aids in the breakdown of fats and the removal of waste from the liver. Some studies suggest that dandelion extract may protect against liver damage caused by oxidative stress and inflammation.

2. Digestive Aid: Dandelion tea is believed to have mild laxative effects, which can help promote healthy digestion and alleviate constipation. It may also stimulate appetite and support overall digestive health by promoting the production of digestive juices.

3. **Diuretic characteristics:** Dandelion tea stimulates the production of urine due to its diuretic characteristics. This may lessen bloating and water retention by helping the body eliminate toxins and extra fluids. However, before using dandelion tea as a diuretic, those with kidney issues should speak with a healthcare provider.

4. **Antioxidant Content:** The flavonoids, phenolic chemicals, and vitamin C found in dandelion aid in the body's fight against oxidative stress and inflammation. These antioxidants may lower the risk of chronic illnesses and shield cells from harm brought on by free radicals.

5. **Possible Blood Sugar Regulation:** Studies on animals have suggested that dandelion extract may help control blood sugar levels and enhance insulin sensitivity. This could be advantageous for those who already have diabetes or are at risk of getting it.

6. Anti-Inflammatory Properties: Compounds in dandelion tea have anti-inflammatory qualities that may help lessen inflammation all throughout the body and soothe the symptoms of illnesses like inflammatory bowel diseases and arthritis.

7. Packed with Nutrients: Vitamin A, C, K, calcium, potassium, iron, and vitamin K are among the many vitamins and minerals that dandelion leaves contain. Increasing your intake of these vital nutrients through the consumption of dandelion tea can promote general health and wellbeing.

It Furthermore, dandelion should be avoided by people who are allergic to other members of the Asteraceae family of plants, which includes ragweed, daisies, and marigolds. Before using dandelion tea in your regimen, as with any herbal therapy, speak with a healthcare provider. This is especially important if you have any underlying medical concerns or are currently taking medication.

Pippali (Long Pepper)

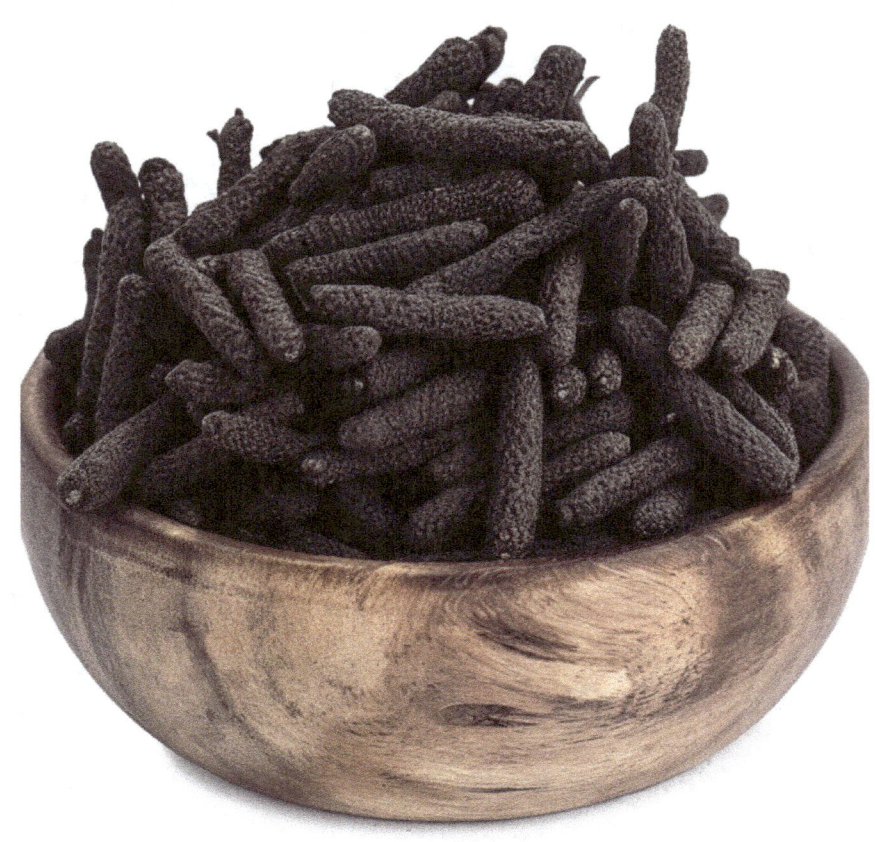

Aids digestion and respiratory health.

Long pepper, or pippali, is a spice that is frequently used in both traditional Ayurvedic medicine and cooking. It comes from the Piper longum plant and is well known for its many health advantages, especially for supporting respiratory and digestive health. Some of its health advantages are as follows:

1. Digestive Aid: It is thought that pippali stimulates the secretion of digestive fluids and enzymes, hence stimulating the digestive system. It can lessen indigestion, enhance appetite, and ease bloating and gas symptoms.

2. **Support for the Respiratory System:** Because of its expectorant qualities, pippali is useful in treating respiratory ailments like asthma, bronchitis, and coughs. It facilitates easier breathing by clearing respiratory tract congestion.

3. Anti-inflammatory: Pippali contains compounds with anti-inflammatory properties, which can help reduce inflammation in the body. This may be particularly useful in conditions like arthritis, where inflammation contributes to joint pain and stiffness

4. **Antioxidant Properties:** The antioxidants in pippali aid in the body's defense against dangerous free radicals, lowering oxidative stress and the chance of developing chronic illnesses including heart disease and some forms of cancer.

5. **Immune Support:** The body's inherent defenses against infections and illnesses can be strengthened by the immune-boosting qualities of pippali.

6. **Weight Management:** Research indicates that pippali may help with weight management by increasing fat metabolism and metabolism. To completely comprehend its impacts in this aspect, more research is necessary.

7. **Increased Nutrient Absorption:** It is thought that pippali increases the nutrients' bioavailability and absorption from diet, which may improve general health and wellbeing.

8. Adaptogenic Properties: Pippali is regarded as an adaptogen, which means that it supports the body's ability to balance and adjust to stress. It might help the body handle stressors that are mental, emotional, and physical.

It is noteworthy that although pippali has been traditionally utilized for its health advantages, further research is necessary to completely understand its modes of action and degree of efficacy in treating different ailments. Furthermore, before adding any new herbs or supplements to your regimen, especially if you are taking medication or have pre-existing health conditions, it is always advisable to speak with a healthcare provider.

Kutki

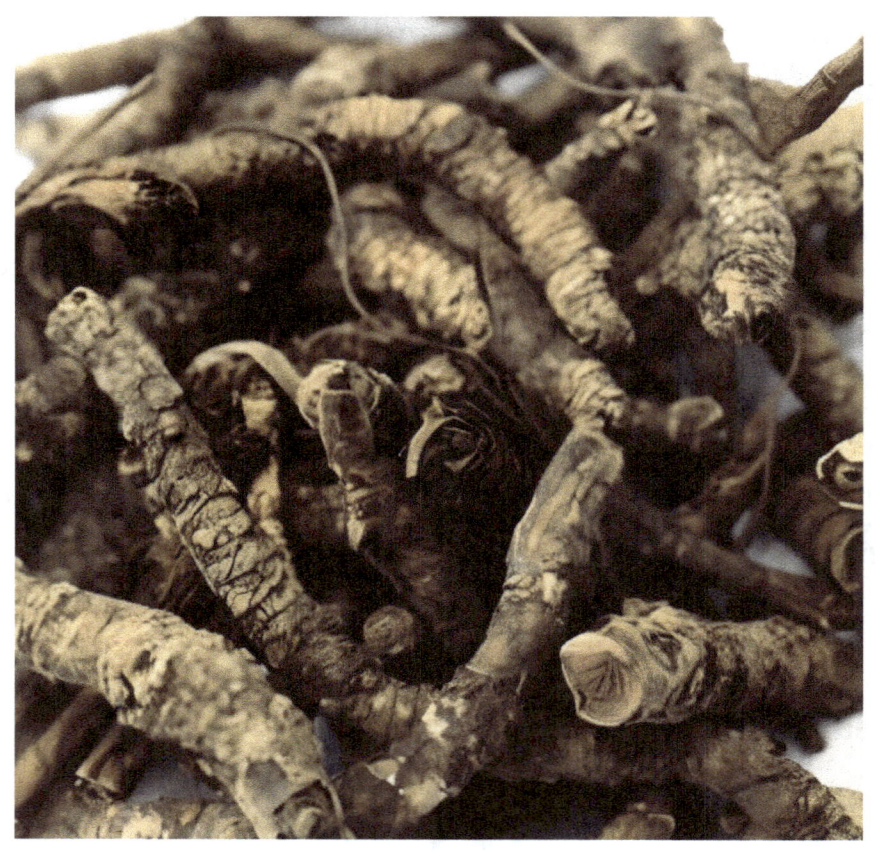

Supports liver function.

Kutki, or Picrorhiza kurroa, is a natural herb of the Himalayas, specifically found in Tibet, Bhutan, India, and Nepal. Its many health benefits—especially in promoting liver function—have led traditional Ayurvedic medicine to employ it for millennia. Kutki has several health advantages, some of them are as follows:

1. Liver Support: Kutki's hepatoprotective qualities are its main claim to fame. It aids in shielding the liver from oxidative stress, poisons, and contaminants. Additionally, it might promote general liver health and help with liver cell regeneration.

2. Detoxification: It is thought that the active ingredients in kutki, such as picroside and kutkin, have detoxifying properties for the body.

3. Anti-inflammatory: Kutki exhibits anti-inflammatory properties, which can be beneficial in conditions involving inflammation, such as arthritis, inflammatory bowel diseases, and certain skin disorders.

4. **Antioxidant:** The antioxidants in kutki protect the body from the damaging effects of free radicals and oxidative stress. This could be a factor in its general health-promoting properties, which include liver protection.

5. **Digestive Health:** Kutki has long been utilized to promote digestive well-being. It might facilitate the release of digestive juices, which helps with nutrition absorption, and help with better digestion and indigestion symptoms.

6. **Immune Support:** According to certain research, kutki may have immunomodulatory effects, which means it may help control how the immune system reacts. This characteristic might help strengthen the body's defenses against illnesses and infections.

7. **Antimicrobial:** Kutki has shown antimicrobial activity against various pathogens, including bacteria, viruses, and fungi. This property may contribute to its traditional use in treating infections and promoting overall immune health.

It is noteworthy that although kutki presents a plethora of potential health benefits, further research is necessary to completely comprehend its modes of action and efficacy in different medical situations. In order to prevent potential interactions or negative effects, it is also imperative that you speak with a healthcare provider before using Kutki, just like you should with any herbal supplement. This is especially true if you have any underlying medical issues or are on medication.

Bilva (Bael)

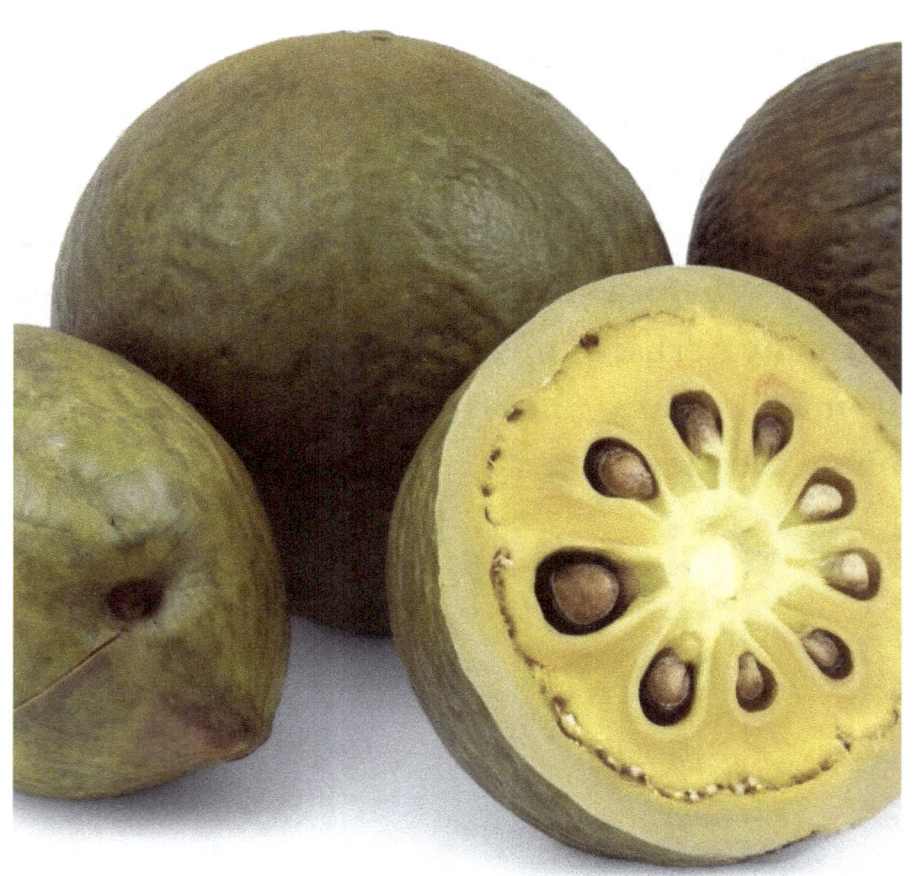

Supports digestive health.

Native to India and Southeast Asia, bilva is sometimes called Bael or Aegle marmelos. Its various health benefits, especially for digestive health, have led traditional medicine systems like Ayurveda to employ it for millennia. The following are a few health advantages of bilva:

1. Digestive Health: The benefits of bilva in supporting digestive health are well known. It is frequently used to treat a variety of gastrointestinal conditions, including constipation, dysentery, and diarrhea. Anti-inflammatory, antibacterial, and laxative chemicals found in the fruit aid in the relief of digestive problems.

2. Treatment for Irritable stool Syndrome (IBS): Traditionally, bilva has been used to ease the symptoms of IBS, including bloating, irregular stool movements, and stomach pain.

3. Relief from Indigestion: Consuming Bilva fruit or its juice is believed to aid digestion and alleviate symptoms of indigestion. It can help in reducing bloating, gas, and discomfort associated with indigestion.

4. Increases Metabolism: Rich in fiber, vitamins, and minerals, bilva has the potential to increase metabolism. This can enhance general metabolic health and help with weight management.

5. Rich in Antioxidants: Antioxidants like vitamin C, which scavenge free radicals and lessen oxidative stress in the body, are present in good amounts in the fruit. This characteristic might improve general health and wellbeing.

6. Cardiovascular Health: By lowering blood pressure and controlling cholesterol, bilva may contribute to the maintenance of cardiovascular health. It is believed that the anti-inflammatory and antioxidant qualities of this substance are good for heart health.

7. Support for the immunological System: The vitamins and minerals in bilva fruit help the body fend against infections and illnesses by boosting immunological function.

8. Skin Health: Because bilva has anti-inflammatory and antibacterial qualities, several traditional remedies recommend using bilva extracts or paste to treat skin diseases like eczema, acne, and rashes.

9. Health of the Respiratory System: Bilva is also utilized in Ayurveda to treat respiratory issues like bronchitis, asthma, and cough. Its expectorant qualities might aid in cleaning the respiratory passages and thinning mucus.

10. Urinary Tract Health: Because bilva is a proven diuretic, it can help flush out toxins and prevent urinary tract infections, which can help promote urinary tract health.

While bilva has many health benefits, it's important to remember that you should always speak with a healthcare provider before adding bilva to your diet, particularly if you have any underlying medical conditions or are taking medication.

Kalmegh

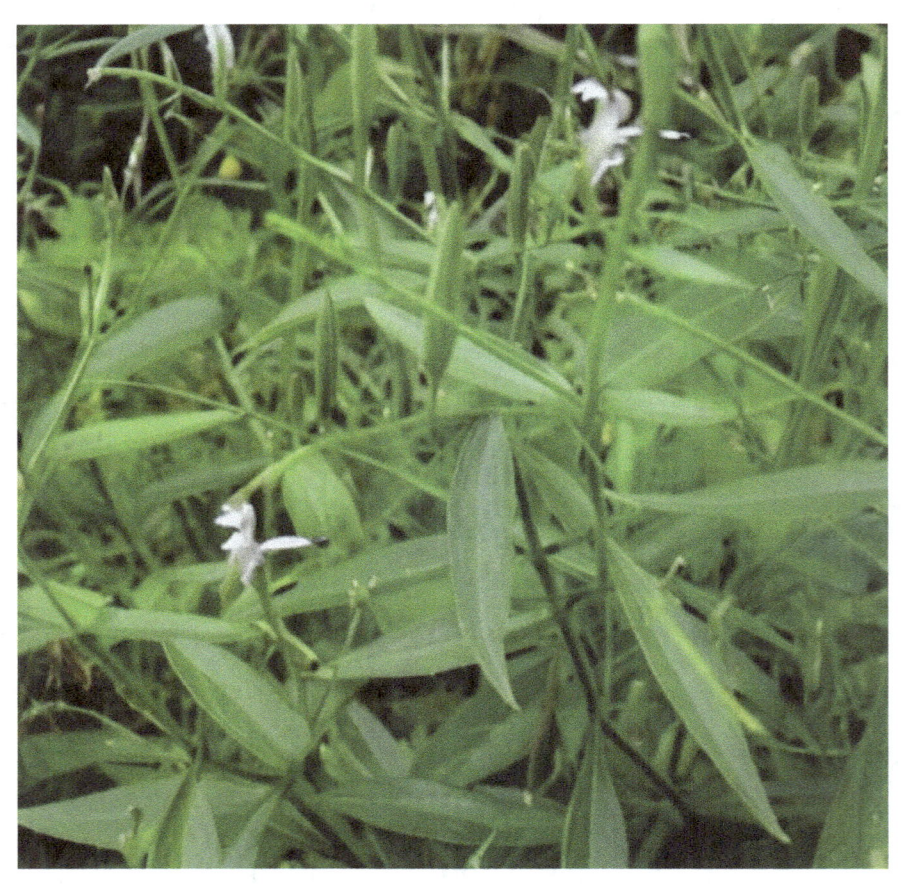

Supports liver health.

Andrographis paniculata, commonly referred to as kalmegh, is a native of South Asian nations including India and Sri Lanka. Because of its many health benefits, it has been utilized for millennia in traditional medical systems such as Ayurveda and Traditional Chinese Medicine. The following are some possible health advantages of kummelgh, especially about liver health support:

1. Liver Protection: Andrographolides, one of the substances found in Kalmegh, has hepatoprotective qualities. These substances aid in shielding the liver from harm brought on by pollution, poisons, and free radicals.

2. Antioxidant Activity: Kalmegh's antioxidants work to scavenge dangerous free radicals from the body, lessening oxidative stress on the liver and improving liver function in general.

3. anti-inflammatory Effects: Kalmegh exhibits anti-inflammatory properties, which can help reduce inflammation in the liver and prevent conditions like hepatitis.

4. Stimulates Bile Production: It is well known that kalmegh causes the liver to produce more bile, which facilitates fat breakdown and aids in digestion.

5. The liver is the main organ in charge of the body's detoxification process. By improving the liver's performance and encouraging the body to rid itself of toxins, kalmegh aids in the detoxification process.

6. Boosts Immunity: Kalmegh is thought to possess immunomodulatory qualities, which means it can aid in immune system regulation. Liver health is one aspect of general health that depends on a functioning immune system.

7. Antiviral and Antimicrobial Properties: Research indicates that Kalmegh may possess antiviral and antimicrobial qualities. These qualities may prove advantageous in the management and prevention of illnesses affecting the liver, such as hepatitis.

8. Supports Liver Regeneration: Kalmegh has the potential to aid in the repair of injured tissues, encourage the growth of new liver cells, and improve liver health in general.

It is noteworthy that although Kalmegh exhibits potential in promoting liver health, further investigation is necessary to completely comprehend its modes of action and effectiveness in managing ailments linked to the liver. Furthermore, before using Kalmegh or any other herbal product, you should always speak with a healthcare provider, particularly if you have a pre-existing medical condition or are on medication.

Mustard Oil (Sarson Tel)

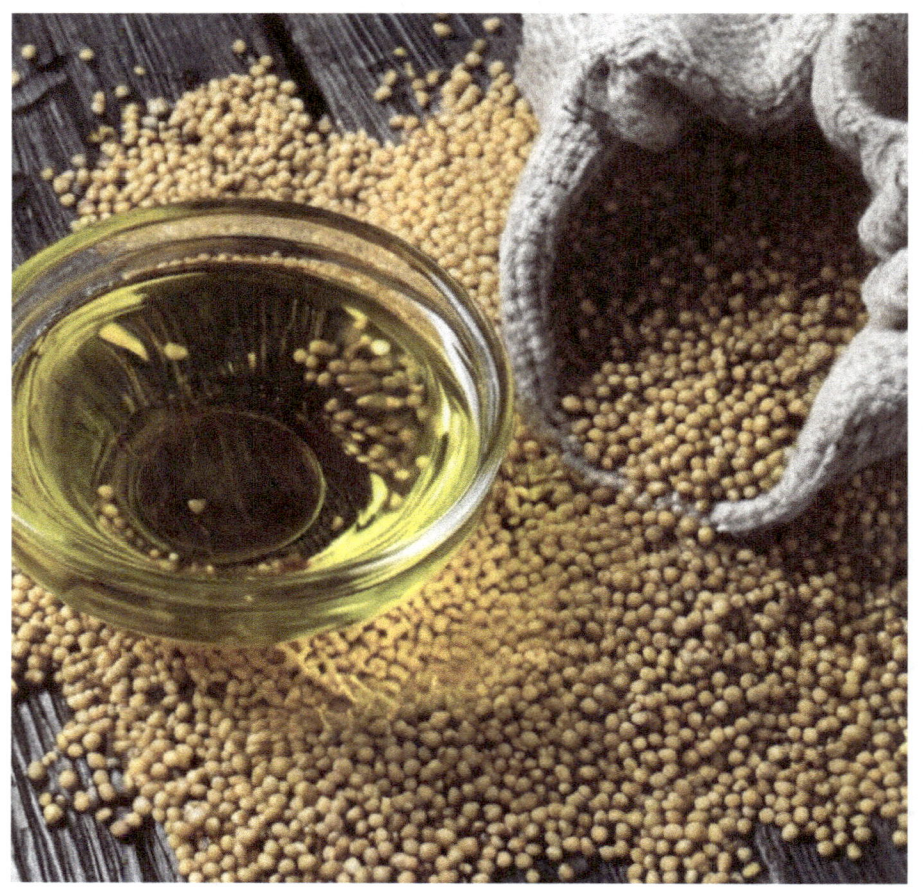

Used in cooking and for massage.

Sarson Tel, another name for mustard oil, is a common cooking oil throughout the world, particularly in South Asia. It is taken out of the mustard plant's (Brassica juncea) seeds by pressing or grinding them. In addition to being used for cooking, mustard oil can also be applied topically, such as in massage therapy. Some of its health advantages are as follows:

1. Rich in Monounsaturated and Polyunsaturated Fats: Both types of fats are thought to be heart-healthy and are abundant in mustard oil. These fats can help lower blood levels of LDL cholesterol, or bad cholesterol, which lowers the risk of heart disease.

2. Source of Omega-3 Fatty Acids: Mustard oil contains a good amount of omega-3 fatty acids, which have anti-inflammatory properties and are essential for brain health, heart health, and overall well-being.

3. Antioxidant Properties: Vitamin E, which helps shield cells from damage brought on by free radicals, is one of the many antioxidants found in mustard oil. Reduced oxidative stress and a decreased risk of chronic illnesses like cancer and heart disease are two benefits of antioxidants.

4. antibacterial and Antifungal effects: Because of substances such as allyl isothiocyanate, mustard oil has antibacterial and antifungal effects. Because of this, it is efficient in warding off germs, fungus, and other infections, improving immunity and general health.

5. Health of the Skin and Hair: Mustard oil can nourish the skin and hair when applied topically. It has minerals and vitamins that hydrate skin, lessen irritation, and encourage hair development. It is said that massaging with mustard oil may increase blood flow and reduce stiffness and soreness in the muscles.

6. **Digestive Health:** By boosting the production of bile and digestive fluids, mustard oil promotes better digestion. Digestive problems such as gas, bloating, and constipation may be lessened by it.

7. **Possible Anti-Inflammatory Effects:** Studies have indicated that mustard oil may have anti-inflammatory qualities, which may help treat ailments including asthma and arthritis.

While mustard oil has several health advantages, it's crucial to remember that moderation is necessary, particularly while cooking. Because of the high potential for injury associated with erucic acid, excessive ingestion may not be advised. Furthermore, because mustard oil has a low smoke point, it should be used with caution while cooking at high heat. Before making big changes to any diet or health-related regimen, it's best to speak with a healthcare provider.

Kesar (Saffron)

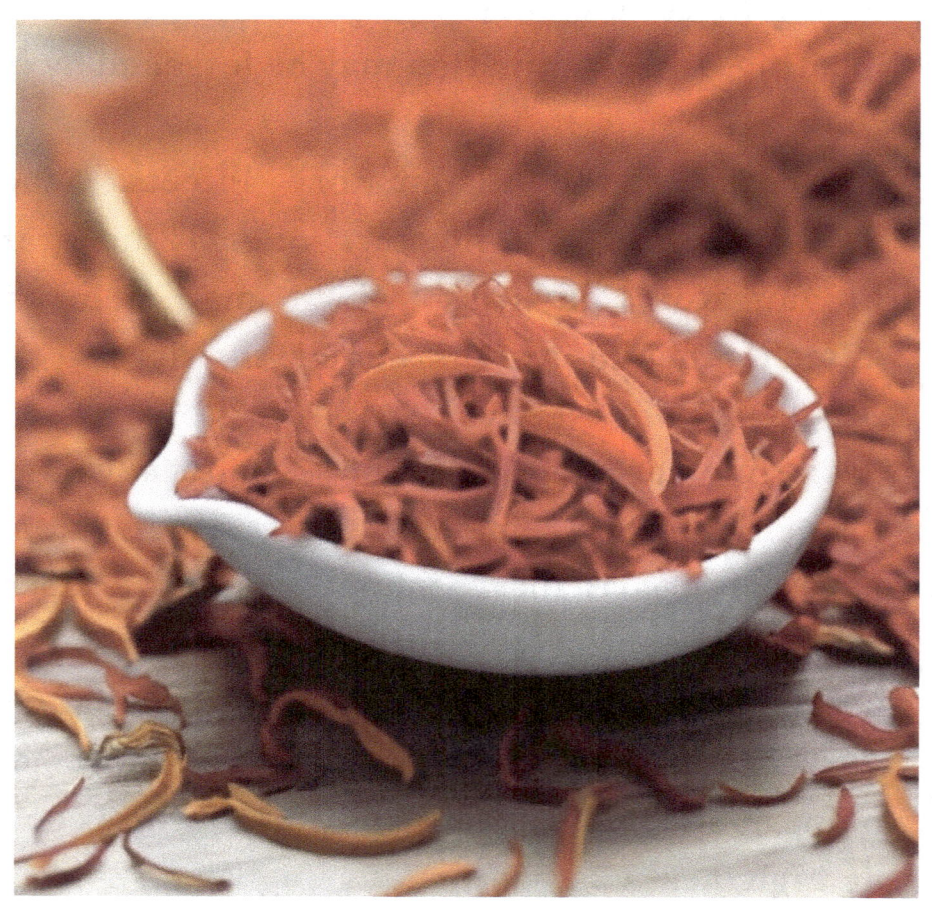

Supports skin health and mood.

Kesar, sometimes referred to as saffron, is a spice made from the blossom of the saffron crocus, or Crocus sativus. The main reason it is grown is for its stigma, which are dried and added to meals as flavoring and coloring. For millennia, saffron has been utilized in many civilizations for its culinary, therapeutic, and medical qualities. Saffron has several health advantages, some of which are as follows:

1. Antioxidant Properties: Strong antioxidants like safranal, crocin, and crocetin are found in saffron. These substances aid in the body's defense against dangerous free radicals, lowering oxidative stress and shielding cells from harm.

2. Mood Enhancement: Saffron has been traditionally used as a natural remedy for improving mood and alleviating symptoms of depression and anxiety. Several studies suggest that saffron may have antidepressant properties and can help in promoting feelings of well-being and relaxation.

3. **Promotes Skin Health:** Due to its anti-inflammatory and antibacterial qualities, saffron is good for keeping skin healthy. In skincare products, it's frequently used to treat acne, lighten blemishes and scars, and encourage a glowing complexion.

4. **Encourages Digestive Health:** In traditional medicine, saffron has been used to ease gastrointestinal discomfort and promote better digestion. It might lessen gas, bloating, and indigestion symptoms.

5. **Possible Anti-Cancer Effects:** Research has indicated that saffron and its bioactive components may possess anticancer qualities, preventing the proliferation of cancer cells and triggering apoptosis, or planned cell death, in a number of cancer kinds.

6. **Improves Cognitive Function:** Research suggests that saffron may have neuroprotective effects and can improve cognitive function. It may help in enhancing memory, concentration, and learning ability, as well as reducing the risk of age-related cognitive decline.

7. Controls Blood Sugar Levels: By increasing insulin sensitivity and decreasing insulin resistance, saffron may assist in controlling blood sugar levels. For those who already have diabetes or are at risk of getting it, this may be advantageous.

8. Aphrodisiac Properties: Saffron has long been believed to have aphrodisiac properties, improving sexual performance and libido. There isn't much scientific data to back up this assertion, although some research indicates that saffron may improve sexual function and health.

It's crucial to remember that, despite the fact that saffron has many health advantages, too much of it might have negative effects. Furthermore, saffron should not be consumed in excess by pregnant women since it may induce uterine contractions.

Manjistha

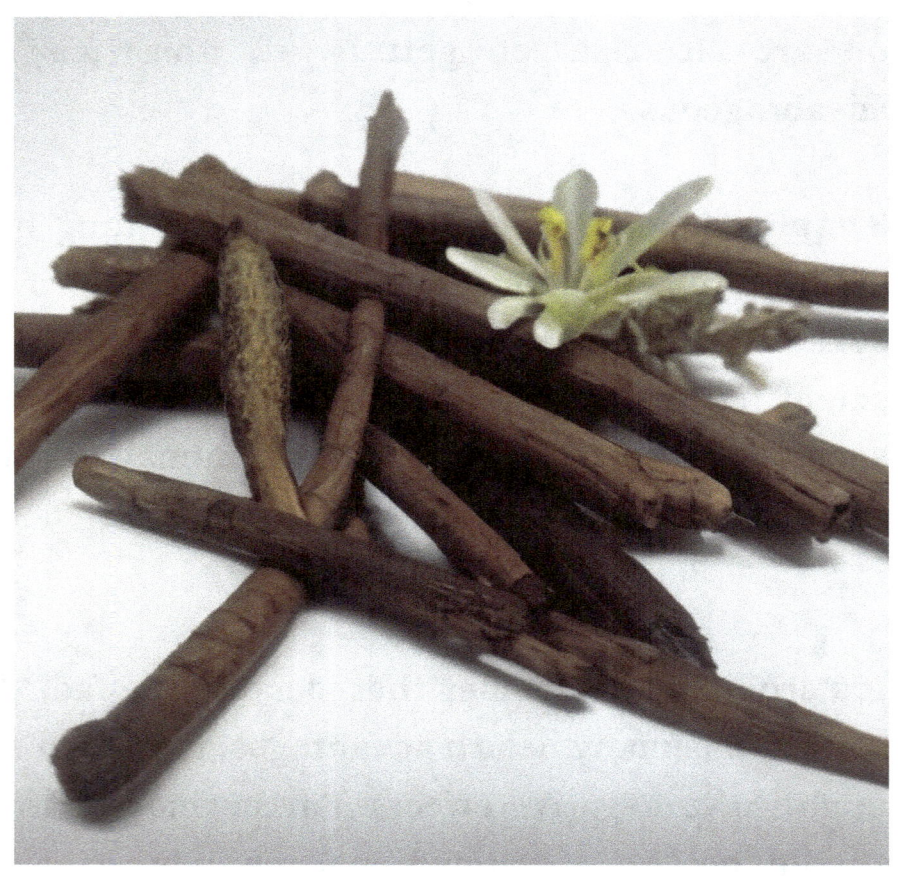

Supports detoxification and skin health.

Manjistha, or Rubia cordifolia in scientific parlance, is a popular herb in Ayurvedic treatment. Its capacity to support skin health and aid in detoxifying are its main claims to fame. Some of its health advantages are as follows:

1. Detoxification: According to Ayurveda, manjistha is a potent blood purifier. It aids in the body's removal of toxins, particularly those from the lymphatic and blood systems. Manjistha can aid the body's natural detoxification processes when taken regularly.

2. Skin Health: Using manjistha regularly can help with skin health. It is said to have antibacterial and anti-inflammatory qualities that can aid in the treatment of several skin disorders, including psoriasis, eczema, and acne. Additionally, manjistha may aid in maintaining a clear complexion and lessening the visibility of imperfections.

3. **Anti-inflammatory:** Compounds in manjistha have anti-inflammatory qualities. It might aid in lessening bodily inflammation, which is advantageous for ailments like inflammatory skin illnesses, joint pain, and arthritis.

4. **Antioxidant:** The herb's abundance of antioxidants aids in the body's defense against dangerous free radicals. Antioxidants are essential for preventing oxidative stress-induced cell damage, which lowers the chance of developing several chronic illnesses and improves general health.

5. **Enhances Liver Health:** It is thought that manjistha enhances liver detoxification and liver function. It might support liver health and prevent diseases linked to the liver by assisting in the liver's detoxification.

6. Supports the Lymphatic System: Manjistha is known to support the lymphatic system, which plays a crucial role in immune function and detoxification.

It might support liver health and prevent diseases linked to the liver by assisting in the liver's detoxification.

7. Diuretic Properties: Manjistha has the ability to promote the production of urine and aid in the body's removal of waste products and excess fluids. Those who struggle with urinary tract infections or fluid retention may find this feature helpful.

8. Promotes Digestive Health: One of manjistha's traditional applications is to promote digestive health. It might aid with constipation relief, better digestion, and gastrointestinal health in general.

Manjistha has several potential health benefits, but individual responses may differ. As always, it's best to speak with a healthcare provider before adding any new herb or supplement to your regimen, especially if you have any underlying medical conditions or are currently taking medication.

Chyawanprash

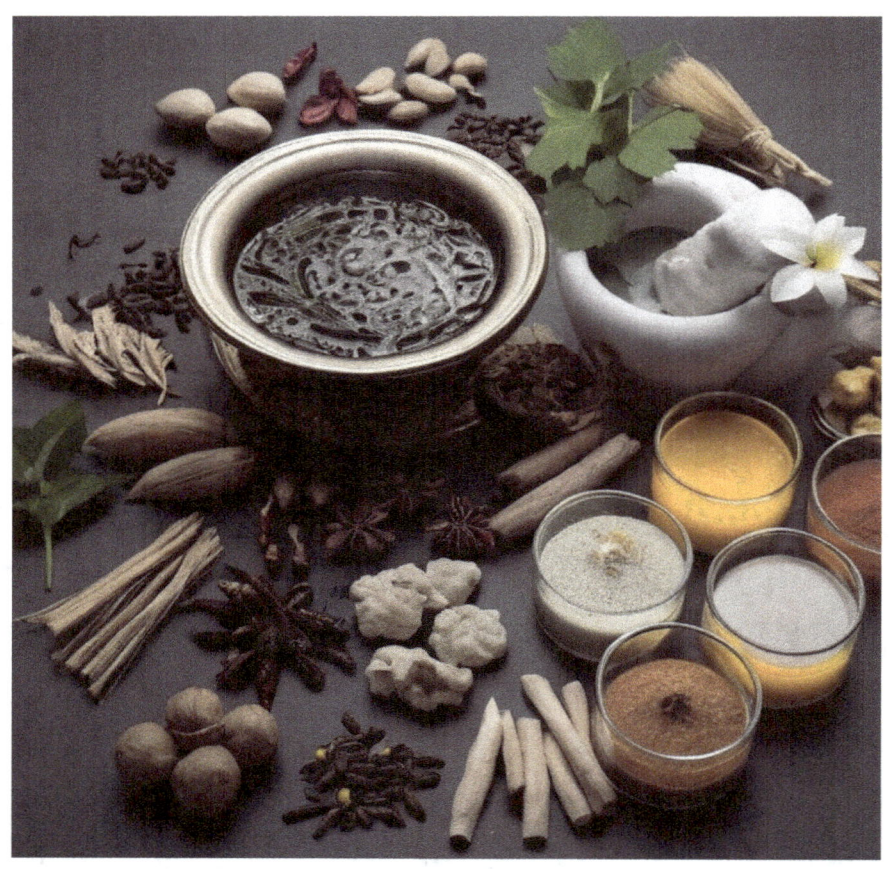

An herbal jam for overall well-being.

For generations, Indians have utilized chyawanprash, a traditional Ayurvedic herbal jam or paste, due to its supposed health benefits. The base component, amla (Indian gooseberry), which is high in vitamin C, is typically combined with other herbs, fruits, spices, and honey. Ashwagandha, ghee (clarified butter), sesame oil, cinnamon, cardamom, and a variety of other herbs and spices are also often used ingredients.

The following are some of the health advantages of chyawanprash:

1. Boosts Immunity: Chyawanprash is thought to fortify the immune system, aiding the body in fending off infections and illnesses, because of its high concentration of Vitamin C from amla and other herbs.

2. Antioxidant Properties: The herbs and spices in Chyawanprash are rich in antioxidants, which help neutralize free radicals in the body and reduce oxidative stress, thus promoting overall health and longevity.

3. Enhances Digestion: A number of the components of Chyawanprash, including cinnamon, cardamom, and ginger, are well-known for their ability to aid in digestion. Regularly consuming chyawanprash may facilitate digestion and enhance gut health.

4. Rejuvenates the Body: Chyawanprash is regarded as a Rasayana in Ayurveda, indicating that it possesses renewing qualities. It is thought to support vitality, nourish the body's tissues, and slow down the aging process.

5. Boosts Respiratory System: It is believed that certain herbs in Chyawanprash, such as licorice and tulsi (holy basil), offer respiratory advantages. Frequent ingestion may support the immune system and lessen the symptoms of illnesses like bronchitis and asthma.

6. Enhances Heart Health: It is thought that several of the constituents in Chyawanprash, like arjuna, enhance heart health by strengthening the heart, lowering cholesterol, and increasing circulation.

7. Boosts Levels of Energy: Chyawanprash is regarded as a natural energizer. Its mixture of spices and herbs releases energy gradually, assisting in the fight against exhaustion and fostering general vitality.

8. Enhances Cognitive Function: Brahmi and Shankhpushpi, two of the herbs in Chyawanprash, are traditionally used to enhance cognitive function, including memory and concentration.

9. Stress Reduction: It is said that the adaptogenic herbs in Chyawanprash, such as ashwagandha and Brahmi, can assist the body in adjusting to stress and foster a feeling of peace and well-being.

It is noteworthy that although Chyawanprash has been used extensively in traditional Ayurvedic treatment and many people vouch for its advantages, there has been relatively little scientific research on its effectiveness. Nonetheless, a number of the specific herbs and components in Chyawanprash have been investigated for their potential health advantages, hence corroborating several of the assertions made regarding this herbal jam.

Gokshura

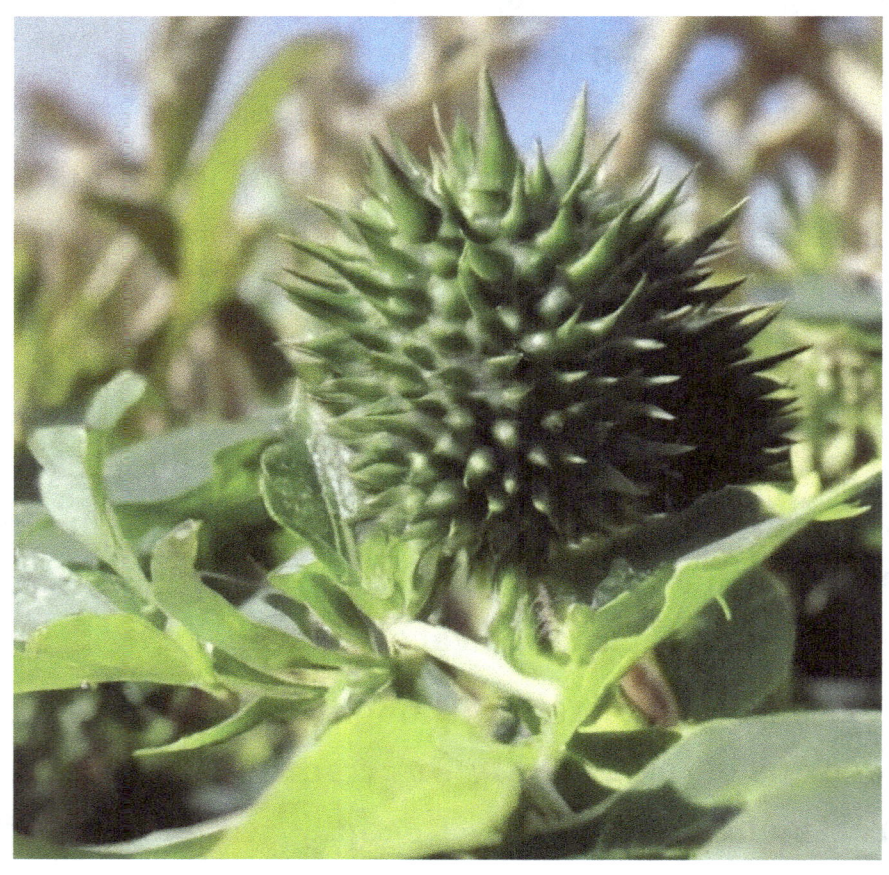

Supports urinary and reproductive health.

Gokshura, botanically known as Tribulus terrestris, is a widely utilized herb in Ayurvedic medicine and other traditional systems of medicine due to its many health advantages, especially in relation to maintaining reproductive and urinary health. Here are a few possible health advantages of it:

1.. Urinary Health: Gokshura is said to have diuretic qualities, which means it could aid in boosting urine production and encouraging the body to rid itself of impurities. Its capacity to improve kidney function is frequently cited as the reason for this activity.

2. Reproductive Health: Gokshura has long been used to promote the reproductive systems of both men and women. It is thought that by promoting healthy testosterone levels in men, it can enhance libido and sexual performance. It may help women with irregular menstruation and promote reproductive health in general.

3. Testosterone Levels: Gokshura is frequently promoted as a natural testosterone enhancer, yet there isn't much scientific proof to back up this assertion. According to certain research, it might aid in raising men's testosterone levels, which might be advantageous for libido, strength, and muscle growth.

4. Antioxidant Properties: Flavonoids, alkaloids, and saponins are just a few of the antioxidants found in gokshura that aid in the body's defense against oxidative stress. This could be a factor in its capacity to support a range of physiological processes and its general health-promoting effects.

5. Athletic Performance: To possibly improve performance and muscle strength, several fitness enthusiasts and athletes take Gokshura supplements. Although there is little scientific proof to support this particular use, it is thought that its possible impacts on energy metabolism and testosterone levels could help athletes perform better.

6. Anti-inflammatory Effects: Gokshura may have anti-inflammatory qualities that could aid in the body's reduction of inflammation and the relief of symptoms related to inflammatory diseases.

7. Immune Support: Gokshura may have the ability to strengthen the immune system, according to certain studies; however, more investigation is required to prove this.

It's important to remember that while gokshura is usually thought to be safe for the majority of people when taken in recommended dosages, some people may experience adverse effects like gastrointestinal distress or allergic responses. Before using any herbal supplement, as with any other, it's best to speak with a healthcare provider, particularly if you have any underlying medical concerns or are currently taking medication.

Bamboo Rice

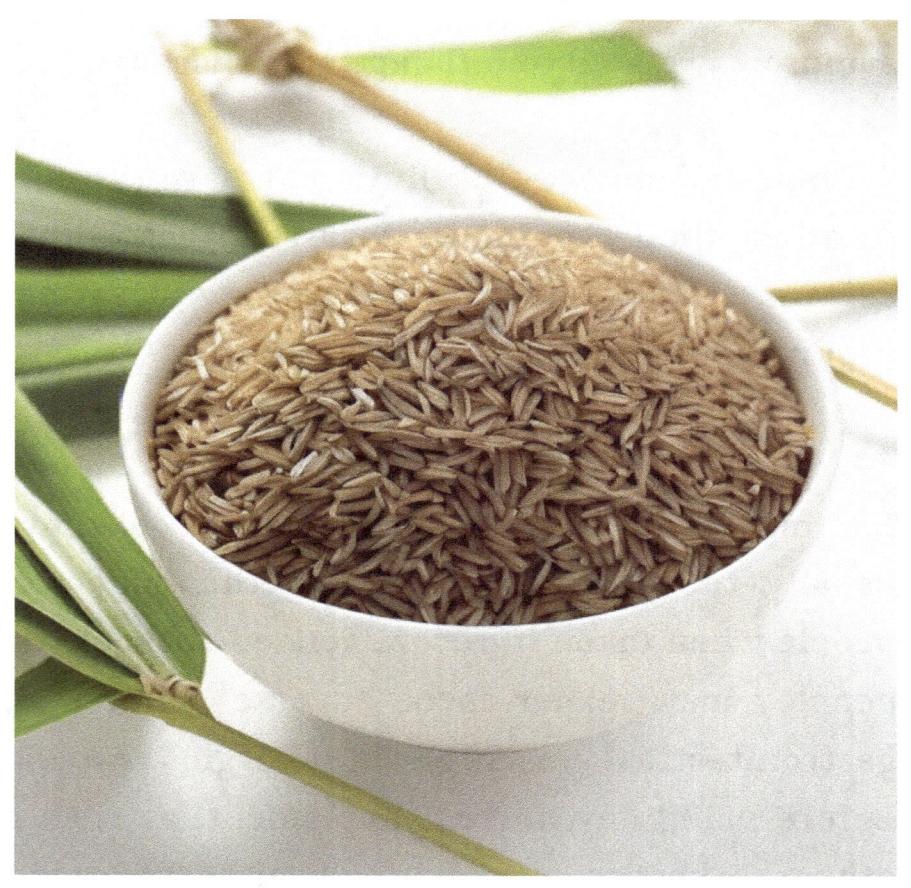

Rich in nutrients, supports overall health.

Bamboo rice is a type of rice that is produced from the seeds of bamboo plants. It is not a separate species of rice but rather a byproduct of the flowering and seeding cycle of certain bamboo species. When bamboo plants reach the end of their life cycle, they produce seeds, and these seeds are then harvested to produce bamboo rice.

Here are some of the health benefits associated with bamboo rice:

1. Nutrient-Rich: Bamboo rice contains various nutrients such as carbohydrates, proteins, fiber, vitamins (especially B vitamins), and minerals (including calcium, magnesium, and manganese). These nutrients are essential for maintaining overall health and well-being.

2. Low Glycemic Index: Bamboo rice has a lower glycemic index compared to regular white rice. Foods with a lower glycemic index release glucose into the bloodstream more slowly, which can help stabilize blood sugar levels and reduce the risk of diabetes and metabolic disorders.

3. Rich in Antioxidants: Flavonoids and phenolic compounds, which are found in bamboo rice, help shield the body from oxidative stress and lower the risk of chronic illnesses like cancer, heart disease, and inflammatory ailments.

4. Digestive Health: The fiber in bamboo rice helps to encourage the growth of good gut bacteria, avoid constipation, and add weight to the stool, all of which contribute to a healthy digestive system. Overall health and the ability to absorb nutrients depend on a functioning digestive tract.

5. Supports Weight Management: Because bamboo rice has a lower glycemic index and more fiber, it can aid in weight management by increasing feelings of fullness, decreasing cravings for food, and controlling appetite. When combined with a balanced diet, it can help those who are trying to reduce or maintain their weight.

6. **Gluten-Free:** Due to its natural lack of gluten, bamboo rice is a good substitute for people who have celiac disease or gluten sensitivity. Those who are on a gluten-free diet can safely consume it.

7. **Energy Booster:** Bamboo rice is a good option for athletes, active people, or anybody else seeking consistent energy throughout the day because of its regular supply of carbohydrates.

8. **Bone Health:** Calcium and magnesium, two elements found in bamboo rice, are critical for strong, healthy bones. Frequent bamboo rice consumption may help lower the risk of bone-related illnesses such as osteoporosis.

Although bamboo rice has many health advantages, it's crucial to remember that in order to get the most out of it, it should be eaten in a balanced diet with other nutrient-dense foods. Individual dietary requirements and preferences should also always be taken into account.

Shankhpushpi

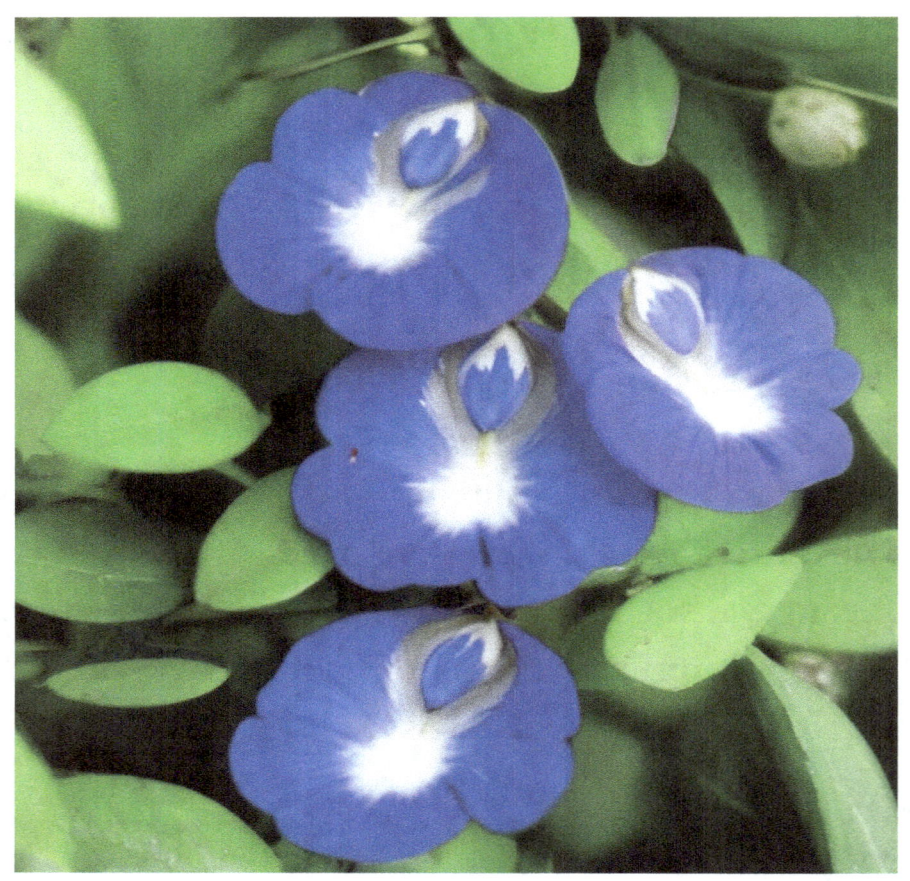

Supports cognitive function and memory.

Convolvulus pluricaulis, also known as sankhpushpi, is a traditional Ayurvedic herb that is well-known for its possible advantages to cognition. Specifically, it is said to help memory and overall brain function. In conventional Indian medical systems such as Ayurveda and Unani, it is frequently used.

The following are some possible health advantages of Shankhpushpi:

1. Memory Improvement: The main benefit of shankhpushpi is its reputation for improving memory and cognitive performance. It might enhance one's capacity for learning and knowledge retention.

2. Stress Reduction: This herb may help the body manage stress better because it is thought to have adaptogenic qualities. It might have a relaxing impact on the neurological system and psyche.

3. **Mental Acuity:** Shankhpushpi is believed to increase alertness and mental clarity. It might facilitate sharper focus and concentration.

4. **Neuroprotective Effects:** According to certain research, shankhpushpi may have neuroprotective qualities that could help shield brain tissue from deterioration and injury.

5. **Antioxidant Activity:** The herb's antioxidant content may be able to lessen the effects of oxidative stress in the brain, which is linked to ageing and neurodegenerative illnesses.

6. **Anxiolytic Effects:** Shankhpushpi is thought to possess anxiolytic (anti-anxiety) effects, which may be a factor in its general ability to soothe and reduce tension.

7. **improved Sleep:** Shankhpushpi is also used in Ayurvedic medicine to alleviate insomnia and encourage improved sleep quality.

It's important to remember that although studies have suggested some possible benefits of Shankhpushpi, which has been utilized for centuries in traditional medicine systems, further research is required to completely understand its mechanisms of action and effectiveness. Before adding Shankhpushpi to your regimen, like with any supplement or herbal therapy, it's best to speak with a healthcare provider, particularly if you have any underlying medical concerns or are on medication.

Punarnava

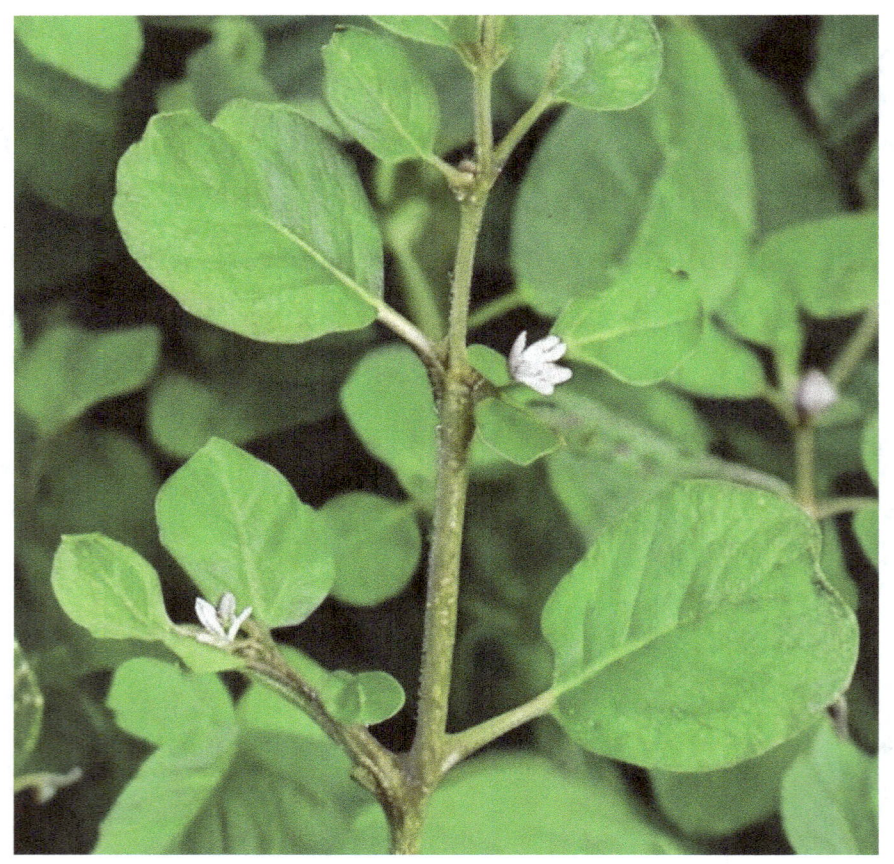

Supports kidney health.

Boerhavia diffusa, another name for the native Indian plant punarva, has been utilized for generations in traditional Ayurvedic medicine. It is thought to offer several health advantages, especially for kidney function. The following are a few possible health advantages of punarva:

1. Kidney Health: The main benefit of punarva is that it increases the output of urine due to its diuretic qualities. As it may aid in the removal of waste materials from the body and help flush out toxins, this may be advantageous for kidney function.

2. UTIs: Punarva is frequently used in Ayurvedic medicine to treat urinary tract infections (UTIs) because of its diuretic and antibacterial qualities. It might aid in lowering inflammation and warding off the bacteria that cause urinary tract infections.

3. Anti-inflammatory Properties: Punarva contains compounds with anti-inflammatory properties, which may help reduce inflammation in the body. This can be beneficial for conditions such as arthritis, gout, and other inflammatory disorders.

4. Punarva has a high antioxidant content, which helps the body counteract dangerous free radicals. Antioxidant activity has the potential to prevent cell damage and lower the risk of chronic illnesses like diabetes, cancer, and cardiovascular disease.

5. Liver Health: According to certain research, punarva may possess hepatoprotective qualities, which means it might aid in preventing harm to the liver. It might help with detoxification procedures and sustain liver function.

6. Heart Health: By assisting in the reduction of blood pressure and cholesterol, punarva may offer advantages for heart health. It may help lessen oxidative stress and inflammation, which may benefit cardiovascular health.

7. Anti-diabetic Effects: Research suggests that Punarva may have hypoglycemic properties, meaning it can help lower blood sugar levels. This could be beneficial for individuals with diabetes or those at risk of developing the condition.

8. Potential to suppress the proliferation of cancer cells is one of the potential anti-cancer qualities of punarva extracts, according to some early research. To completely comprehend its implications in this domain, more research is necessary.

It's crucial to remember that although punarva has been used for a variety of medicinal purposes throughout history and has shown promise in studies, further research is required to completely understand its safety and effectiveness. Before using Punarva, like with any herbal therapy, it is best to speak with a healthcare provider, particularly if you are on medication or have any underlying medical conditions.

Vacha (Sweet Flag)

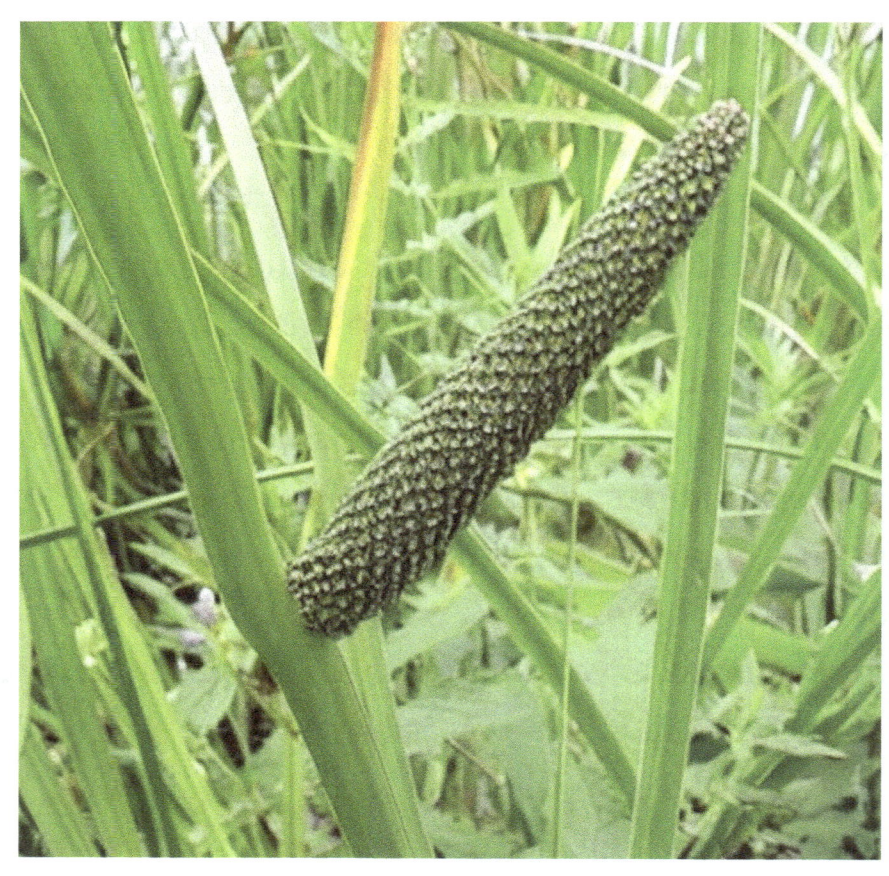

Supports respiratory health.

Vacha, sometimes referred to as Sweet Flag or Acorus calamus, is a perennial herb that has long been utilized in Ayurvedic and other traditional medical systems. Its long, blade-like leaves and fragrant underground stems, known as rhizomes, are what define this native plant of Asia and Europe. Vacha is prized for its therapeutic qualities and is thought to provide a number of health advantages, including promoting respiratory health. Here are a few possible health advantages of it:

1. Vacha is frequently utilized to promote respiratory health. It is thought to contain expectorant qualities, which aid in clearing the respiratory system of congestion and phlegm. For ailments including asthma, bronchitis, and coughs, this may be helpful.

2. Digestive Health: Vacha is thought to aid digestion by stimulating the secretion of digestive juices and enzymes. It may help relieve symptoms of indigestion, bloating, and flatulence.

3. **Support for the Nervous System:** Vacha is an Ayurvedic nervine tonic, which means it helps the nervous system. It is thought to provide relaxing and soothing qualities that can lessen tension, unease, and anxiety.

4. **Memory and Cognitive Function:** Improving memory and cognitive function is one of the traditional applications of vacha. It is thought to enhance mental clarity, focus, and concentration.

5. Vacha is composed of chemicals that have anti-inflammatory qualities. It might help reduce inflammation in different body areas, which could be advantageous for ailments like inflammatory bowel illnesses and arthritis.

6. **Effects against Microbes:** Research has been done on the antibacterial qualities of vacha. Its efficacy in treating respiratory and digestive illnesses may be attributed to its ability to suppress the growth of bacteria, fungus, and viruses.

7. **Effects on Analgesia:** Vacha is thought to possess analgesic (pain-relieving) qualities. It might ease the discomfort associated with toothaches, headaches, and other ailments.

8. **Enhances Appetite:** Vacha is beneficial for people who have poor digestion or appetite loss because it is believed to enhance appetite.

Vacha has several possible health benefits, but because it includes several substances that can be dangerous in excessive doses, it must be used carefully and under the supervision of a skilled healthcare professional. Children, women who are breastfeeding or pregnant, and anyone who have specific medical concerns should not use Vacha without first speaking with a healthcare provider. Additionally, in order to guarantee the quality and safety of Vacha, it is imperative that you get it from reliable vendors.

Khadira

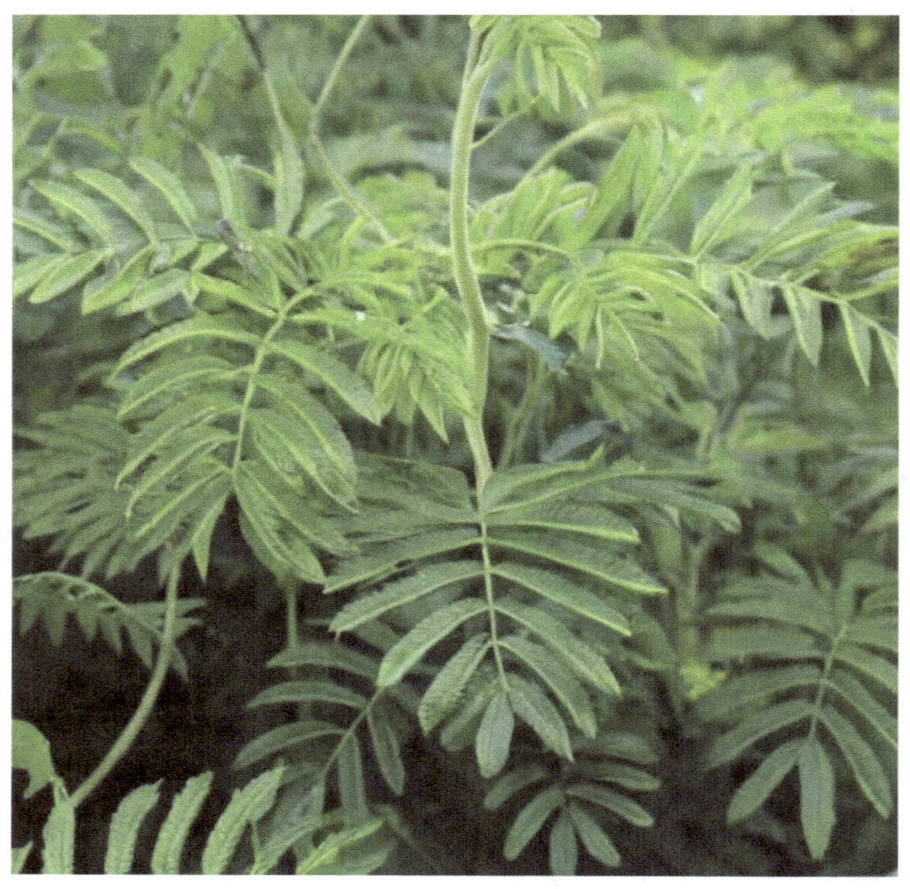

Supports oral health.

Acacia catechu, also referred to as khadira, is a native South and Southeast Asian medicinal shrub. It has long been utilized in Ayurvedic medicine for its many health advantages, one of which being promoting dental health. The following are a few possible health advantages of Khadira:

1. Oral Health: Khadira's astringent qualities can aid in gum tightening and the prevention of gum conditions like gingivitis. Because it can combat oral bacteria and plaque, it is frequently found in mouthwash and toothpaste products.

2. Anti-Inflammatory Properties: Khadira has anti-inflammatory components in it. It might aid in lessening digestive tract, throat, and mouth irritation.

3. Antimicrobial Effects: The antimicrobial properties of Khadira make it effective against various bacteria, fungi, and viruses. It can help prevent infections in the mouth and throat.

4. **Wound Healing:** Khadira has been traditionally used topically to aid in wound healing. Its astringent properties help in tightening the skin and reducing bleeding.

5. **Antioxidant Activity:** Khadira contains antioxidants that help protect cells from damage caused by free radicals. This may have a positive effect on overall health and well-being.

6. **Digestive Health:** Some traditional uses of Khadira involve its use in treating digestive issues such as diarrhea and dysentery. Its antimicrobial properties may help combat the pathogens responsible for these conditions.

7. **Skin Health:** Because of its astringent and antibacterial qualities, Khadira is also utilized in a number of skincare products. It might aid with acne treatment, lessen excessive oiliness, and enhance the general health of the skin.

8. Blood Sugar Regulation: Some research suggests that Khadira may have hypoglycemic effects, meaning it could help lower blood sugar levels. This property might be beneficial for individuals with diabetes or those at risk of developing diabetes.

It's important to note that while Khadira has been used for centuries in traditional medicine systems like Ayurveda, more research is needed to fully understand its mechanisms of action and potential side effects.

Bael Juice

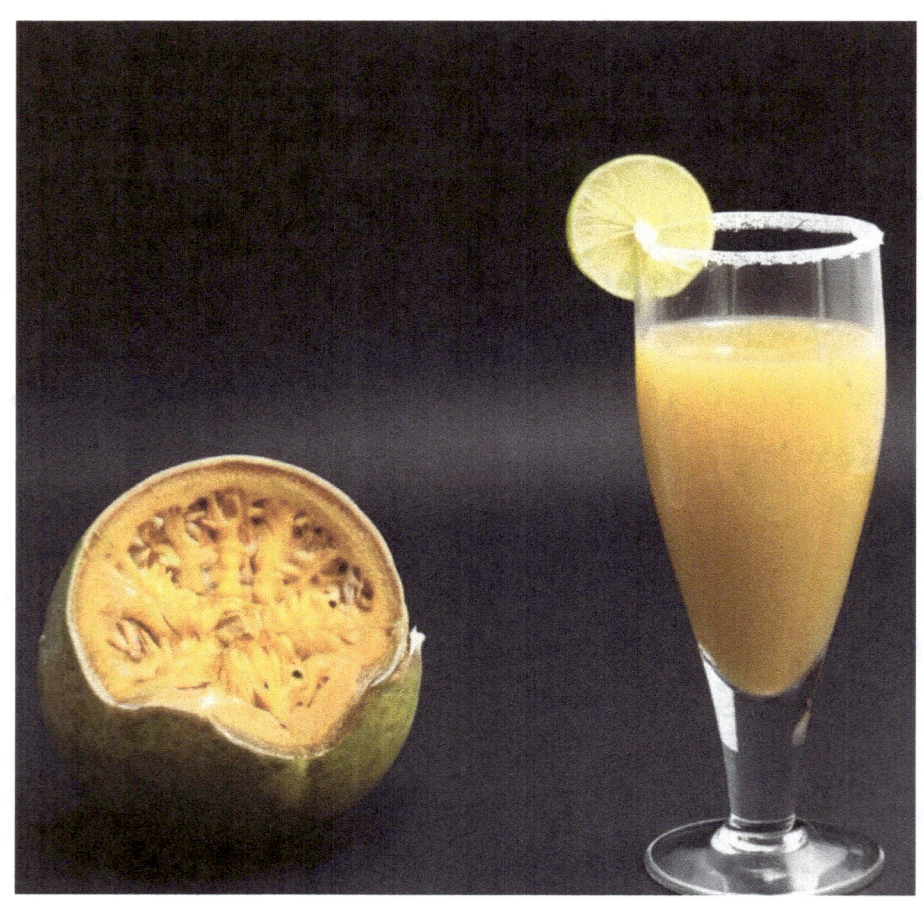

Supports digestive health.

The pulp of the bael fruit, often called wood apple (Aegle marmelos), is used to make bael juice. It is well-liked throughout Asia, but especially in India, where people appreciate it for possible health advantages. The following are some health advantages of bael juice, especially in terms of promoting digestive health:

1. Relieves Constipation: The laxative qualities of bael juice are well known for their ability to relieve constipation. Bael fruit's high fiber content facilitates easy digestion and aids in the regulation of bowel motions.

2. Treats Diarrhea: Bael juice has a laxative effect, but it also has some benefits for treating diarrhea. The fruit's tannins aid in keeping loose stools together, which relieves diarrhea.

3. Soothes Digestive Issues: Bael juice possesses anti-inflammatory properties that can help soothe various digestive issues such as indigestion, acidity, and gastritis. It helps in reducing inflammation in the gastrointestinal tract, thereby providing relief from discomfort.

4. Enhances Digestive Process: By encouraging the secretion of digestive enzymes, regular bael juice ingestion may enhance digestive process overall. Better digestion may result from this assistance in the breakdown and absorption of nutrients from meals.

5. Enhances Gut Health: The components in betel juice encourage the development of good gut bacteria, which are critical for keeping the digestive tract in good condition. Having a balanced gut flora is essential for good digestion and general health.

6. Rich in Nutrients: Bael fruit is a good source of calcium, potassium, and magnesium in addition to important vitamins A, C, and B complex. These minerals promote overall vitality and help with many digestive health issues.

7. Hydrating: Bael juice has a high water content, which helps keep the body hydrated. Proper hydration is essential for maintaining optimal digestive function and preventing issues like constipation.

It's important to note that while bael juice offers potential health benefits, individuals with certain medical conditions or allergies should consult with a healthcare professional before incorporating it into their diet. Additionally, moderation is key, as excessive consumption of bael juice may lead to adverse effects such as gastrointestinal discomfort.

Kokum

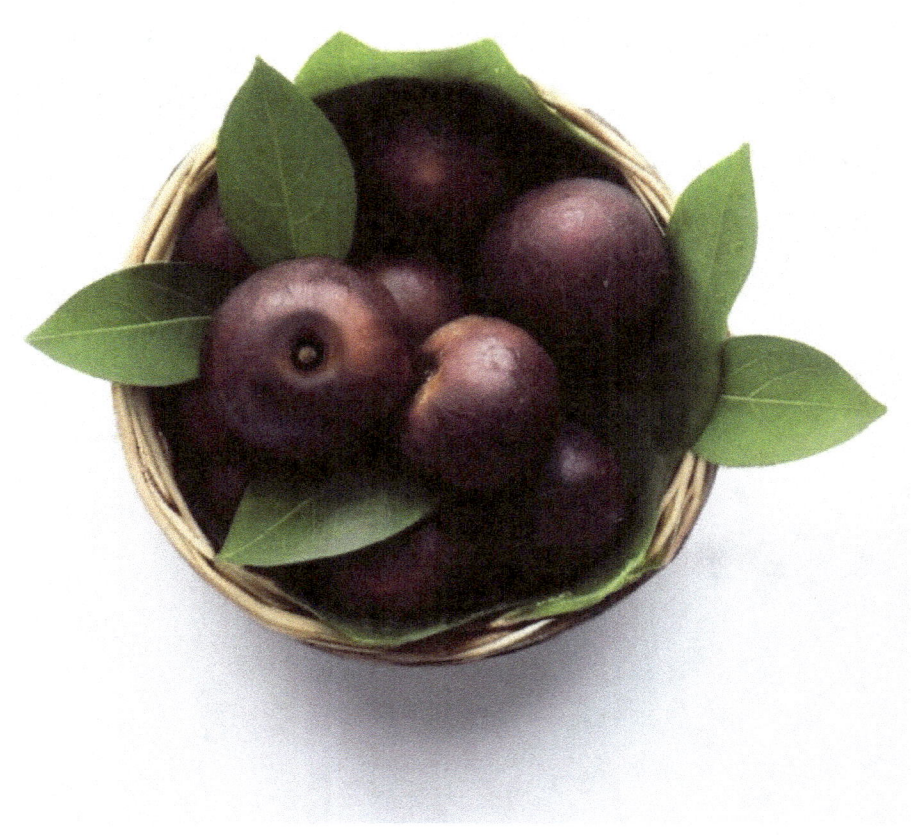

Supports digestion and hydration.

The tropical fruit kokum, also called Garcinia indica, is indigenous to India's Western Ghats. Indian food is used it extensively, especially in states like Maharashtra, Karnataka, and Goa. Kokum is well known for its culinary and therapeutic qualities. Some of its health advantages are as follows:

1. Promotes Digestion: The high dietary fiber content of kokum promotes healthy digestion and helps ward against constipation. Additionally, substances like hydroelectricity acid (HCA) are present, which are thought to activate the digestive enzymes and improve digestion.

2. Hydration: Kokum is frequently used to make kokum sherbet, a refreshing beverage. This drink is cooling and aids in maintaining bodily fluids, particularly in the sweltering summer months. As a natural coolant, it is.

3. **Antioxidant Properties:** Rich in xanthones and vitamin C, kokum is an excellent source of antioxidants. By assisting the body in combating free radicals, these substances lessen oxidative stress and the chance of developing chronic illnesses.

4. **Anti-inflammatory:** Kokum has anti-inflammatory qualities since it contains substances like garcinol. It can aid in lowering bodily inflammation and easing the symptoms of illnesses like inflammatory bowel disorders and arthritis.

5. **Weight Control:** According to certain studies, kokum may help in weight control. Kokum contains compounds, such as HCA, that may help reduce hunger and prevent the body from turning carbs into fat, which could support weight loss attempts.

6. **Lowers Cholesterol:** Kokum may have cholesterol-lowering properties due to its fiber content and other bioactive compounds.

Regular consumption of kokum may help maintain healthy cholesterol levels and reduce the risk of heart disease.

7. **Enhances Metabolism:** It is thought that kokum increases metabolism, which can aid in the body's ability to produce energy and better absorb nutrients.

8. **Relieves Gastric Issues:** Acidity, bloating, and flatulence are among the digestive issues that kokum is frequently used to treat. Its calming qualities help ease discomfort and calm the lining of the stomach.

9. **Skin Health:** By preventing free radical damage and encouraging the creation of collagen, the antioxidants in kokum can help to improve the health of the skin. Because of its moisturizing and restorative qualities, kokum butter, which is made from kokum seeds, is utilized in skincare items.

In general, kokum is a great complement to a well-balanced diet and provides several health advantages.

But it's important to use it sparingly and speak with a doctor, particularly if you have any pre-existing medical concerns or are expecting or nursing a child.

Jatamansi

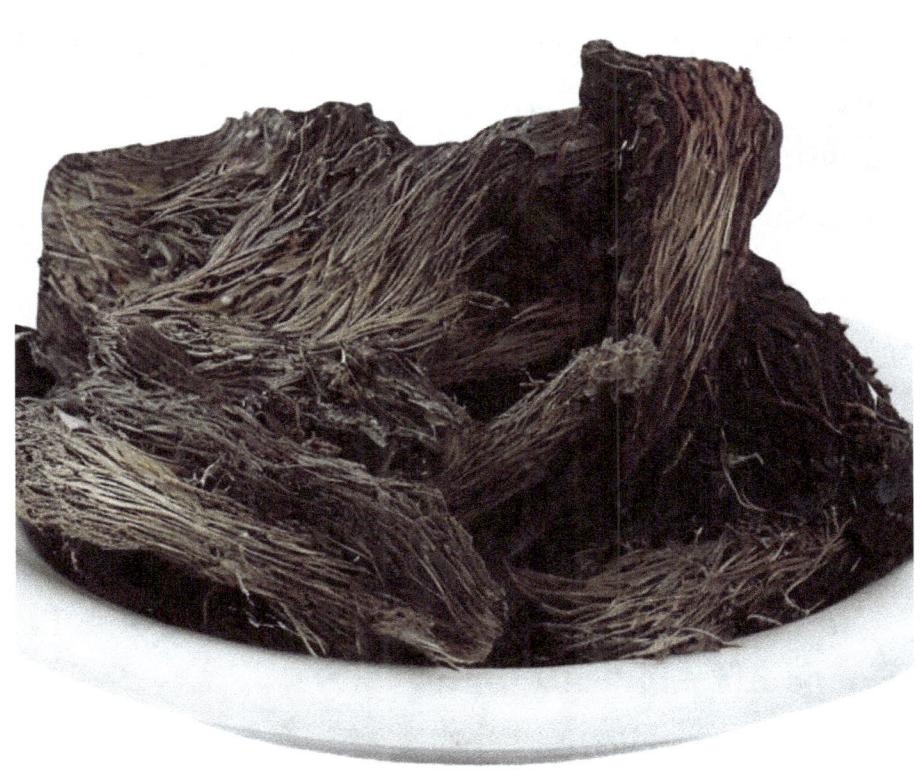

Jatamansi: Calming herb, supports stress management.

The perennial plant jatamansi, also called spikenard or Nardostachys jatamansi, is indigenous to the Himalayan region and is mostly found in China, India, Nepal, and Bhutan. For millennia, Ayurvedic medicine has utilized it for its numerous health advantages, especially its ability to soothe and alleviate tension. The following are a few possible health advantages of jatamansi:

1. Reduction of Stress: Jatamansi is well renowned for its ability to calm and relax people. It's thought to aid in lowering tension, fear, and uneasiness. It might function by restoring the proper balance of brain chemicals linked to mood control, like dopamine and serotonin.

2. Improved Sleep: Due to its calming effects, Jatamansi is often used to promote better sleep quality. It may help individuals suffering from insomnia or other sleep disorders by inducing a sense of relaxation and tranquility.

3. Cognitive Health: According to certain research, jatamansi may possess neuroprotective qualities that could fend against cognitive aging and promote general brain health. Additionally, it might improve focus, memory, and cognitive function.

4. Flavonoids and sesquiterpenes are two examples of the chemicals found in jatamansi that have antioxidant qualities. Antioxidants aid in the body's defense against dangerous free radicals, lowering inflammation and oxidative stress—both of which are linked to several chronic illnesses.

5. Anti-Inflammatory Effects: Jatamansi has long been used to reduce pain and inflammation. It might assist in easing the symptoms of inflammatory diseases such headaches, arthritis, and muscular soreness.

6. Cardiovascular Health: Studies indicate that by assisting in the regulation of blood pressure and cholesterol, jatamansi may have cardioprotective benefits.

It might also improve heart health in general by lowering inflammation and oxidative stress.

7. Digestive Support: Jatamansi is occasionally used in Ayurvedic medicine to support healthy digestion and relieve digestive problems like heartburn, bloating, and gastrointestinal spasms.

8. Skin and Hair Care: Because of its alleged benefits for the skin and hair, jatamansi oil is frequently used topically in skincare and haircare products. Its ability to lower inflammation, ease irritation, and even out skin tone may contribute to the promotion of healthy skin. It is also thought to strengthen hair follicles, nourish the scalp, and stop hair loss.

It is noteworthy that although jatamansi has been used traditionally for a long time and has shown some encouraging findings, further clinical studies are required to completely understand its mechanisms of action and usefulness in treating different illnesses.

Dashmool

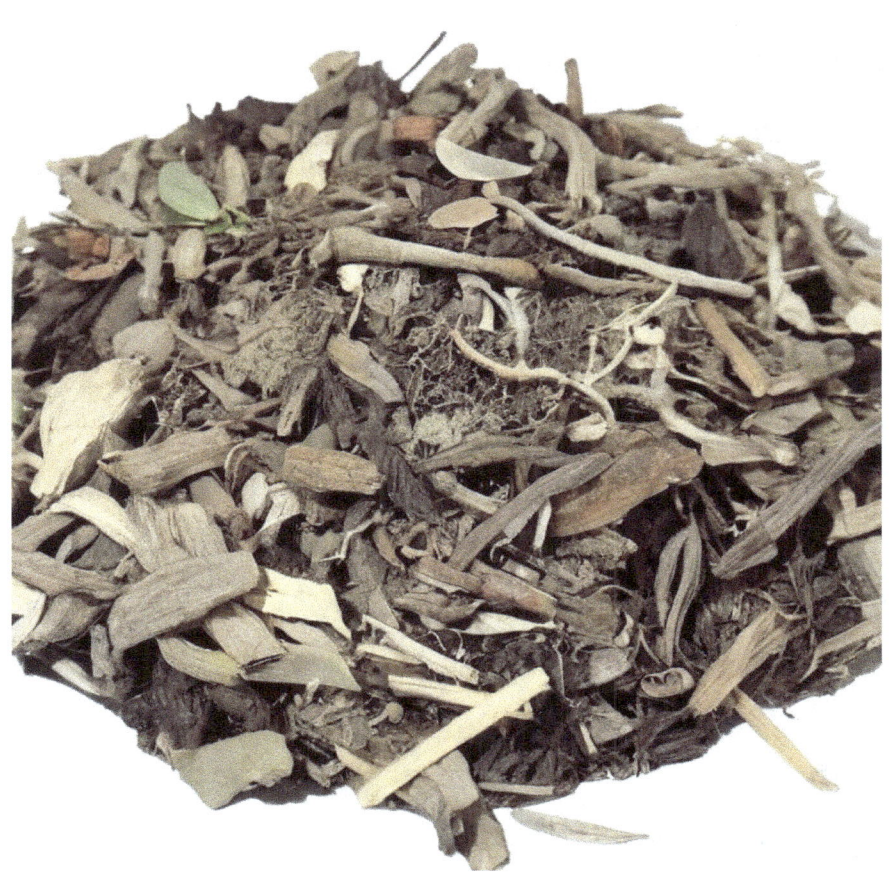

A blend of ten roots for various health benefits.

A traditional Ayurvedic remedy, Dashmool is derived from 10 distinct roots. In Sanskrit, the word "Dashmool" means "ten roots". These roots are carefully chosen and blended to provide a powerful treatment that offers a number of health advantages. Depending on the area and custom, the precise roots used in Dashmool can change slightly, but generally speaking, they consist of:

- Bilva (Aegle marmelos)
- Agnimantha (Premna integrifolia)
-
- Shyonaka (Oroxylum indicum)
- Patala (Stereospermum suaveolens)
- Gambhari (Gmelina arborea)
- Brihati (Solanum indicum)
- Kantakari (Solanum xanthocarpum)
- Shalparni (Desmodium gangeticum)
- Prishnaparni (Uraria picta)
- Gokshura (Tribulus terrestris)

Each of these roots possesses unique medicinal properties, and when combined, they synergistically enhance each other's effects. Some of the potential health benefits of Dashmool include:

1. Anti-inflammatory Properties: Dashmool has long been used to treat illnesses including arthritis, joint pain, and muscular stiffness by reducing inflammation in the body.

2. Analgesic (Pain-Relieving) Effects: Dashmool effectively reduces pain associated with a variety of diseases because of its anti-inflammatory effects.

3. Support for the Respiratory System: Dashmool is known to have bronchodilator qualities, which can aid in the treatment of respiratory conditions like cough, bronchitis, and asthma.

4. Nourishment and Rejuvenation: This mixture is thought to contain nourishing qualities that replenish the body and support general vigor and well-being.

5. Assists with Digestion: Dashmool is used to promote healthy gastrointestinal function, alleviate gas and bloating, and assist with digestion.

6. Nervine Tonic: It is thought to be advantageous for the nervous system, assisting in mental calmness, stress reduction, and relaxation.

7. Promotes Women's Health: Dashmool is frequently suggested for conditions affecting women's health, such as irregular menstruation, postpartum recuperation, and menopausal symptoms.

8. Immune Support: According to certain Ayurvedic practitioners, Dashmool can help bolster the immune system, increasing the body's resistance to illnesses and infections.

9. Support for the Heart and Circulation: According to certain traditional usage, Dashmool may provide advantages for the heart and circulation.

Dashmool has been a part of traditional Ayurvedic medicine for centuries, and while it is generally considered safe when used as directed, it is best to see a qualified healthcare practitioner before using any herbal remedy, particularly if you are taking medication or have underlying health conditions.

Kumari (Aloe Vera Juice)

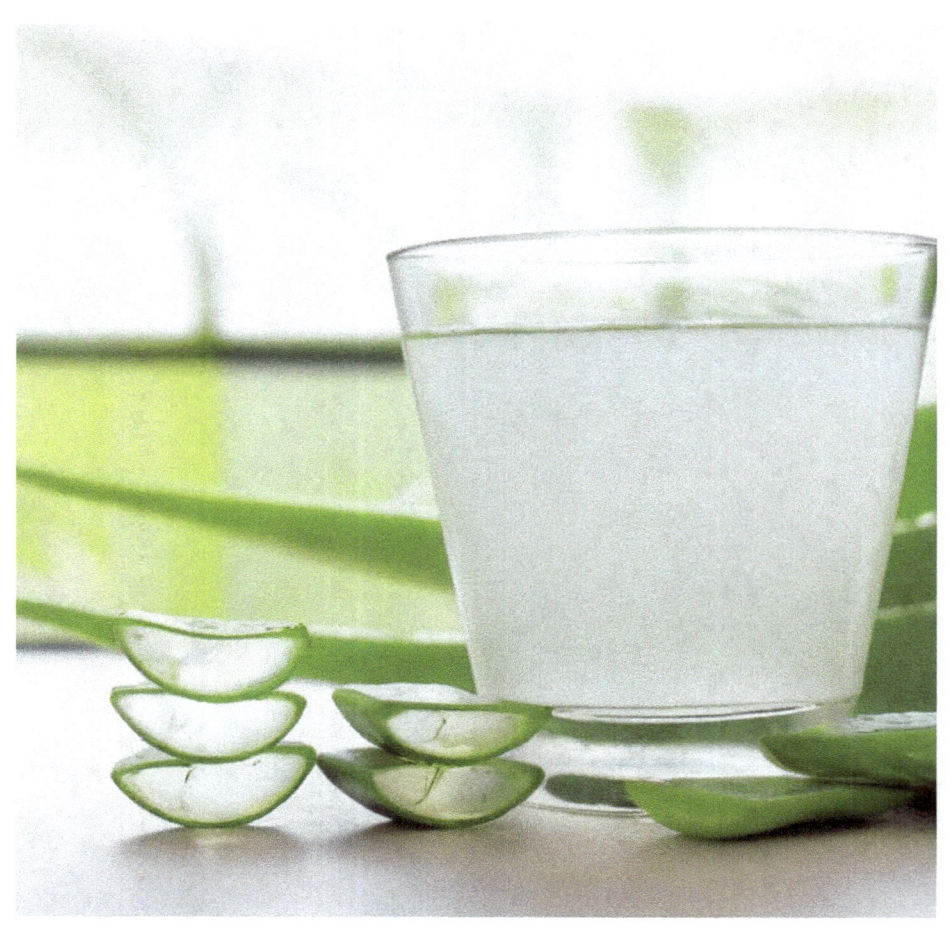

Supports digestion and skin health.

The Aloe Vera plant, which has been utilized for centuries for its therapeutic benefits, is the source of Kumari, sometimes referred to as Aloe Vera juice. Here are a few possible health advantages of it:

1. Digestive Aid: Aloe Vera juice is often used to promote the health of the digestive system. It has ingredients including aloin and aloe-emodin that may help control bowel motions and lessen the symptoms of gastrointestinal conditions like acid reflux and irritable bowel syndrome (IBS).

2. Hydration: Aloe Vera juice is a great source of hydration because of its high water content. Drinking enough water is crucial for sustaining general health and sustaining biological processes.

3. Hydration: Aloe Vera juice is a great source of hydration because of its high water content. Drinking enough water is crucial for sustaining general health and sustaining biological processes.

4. Skin Health: Aloe Vera's advantages for the skin are widely recognized. Its moisturizing qualities and antioxidant, vitamin, and mineral content nourish the skin, aid in healing, and may be beneficial for eczema, psoriasis, and acne.

5. Immune System Support: Because of its antioxidant qualities, some study indicates that aloe vera may help support the immune system. The body uses antioxidants to combat damaging free radicals, which can improve general health and wellness.

6. Weight control: Studies indicate that by enhancing digestion and cleansing the body, aloe vera juice may help with weight management. Nevertheless, additional studies are required to validate these impacts.

While aloe vera juice has many potential health benefits, individual results may differ. As such, it's important to speak with a healthcare provider before using aloe vera juice regularly, particularly if you have any underlying medical conditions or are taking medication.

Yastimadhu (Licorice)

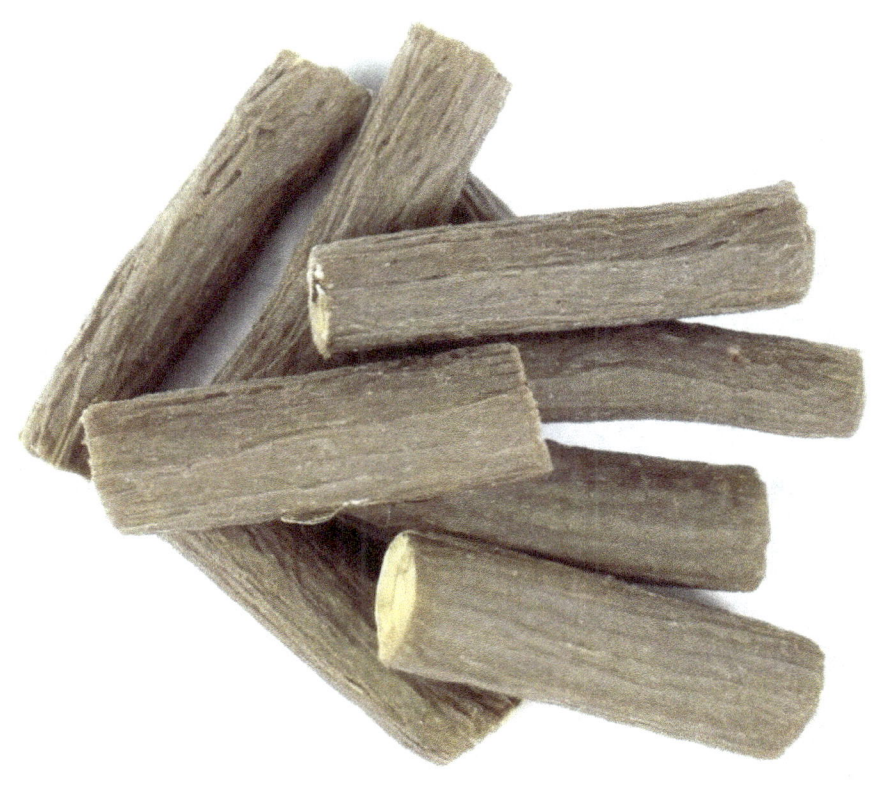

Supports respiratory health.

Yastimadhu, a herbaceous perennial plant native to southern Europe and portions of Asia, is often referred to as licorice or Glycyrrhiza glabra. Because of its many health benefits, the root of the licorice plant is frequently utilized in traditional medical systems such as Ayurveda, Traditional Chinese Medicine (TCM), and Unani medicine. Here are a few possible health advantages of it:

1. Digestive Health: Traditionally, licorice was used to treat gastrointestinal problems like heartburn, indigestion, and stomach ulcers. It is thought to possess anti-inflammatory qualities that could aid in lessening intestinal and stomach inflammation.

2. Health of the Respiratory System: Licorice root is frequently used to treat respiratory issues like bronchitis, sore throats, and coughs. It has ingredients that can aid in clearing congestion and thinning mucus.

3. Anti-inflammatory Properties: Compounds found in licorice, such as glycyrrhizin, have demonstrated anti-inflammatory effects, which may help reduce inflammation in various parts of the body.

4. Support for the Immune System: Antioxidants included in licorice root can strengthen the immune system and shield the body from oxidative stress.

5. Hormonal Balance: The structure of ligorice root's glycyrrhizinic acid is comparable to that of aldosterone, a hormone that controls the balance of sodium and potassium. Traditionally, licorice has been used to assist balance hormones, especially in women going through menopause.

6. Skin Health: Because licorice extract has anti-inflammatory and antioxidant qualities, it's frequently utilized in skincare products. It might lessen redness, ease skin irritations, and brighten dark spots.

6. Cognitive Health: According to some research, licorice contains chemicals that may have neuroprotective properties, which could improve memory and cognitive function.

7. Anti-viral and Anti-bacterial Properties: Studies on licorice have indicated that it may be helpful in the battle against infections by preventing the growth of some viruses and bacteria.

Liver Health: It is thought that licorice root possesses hepatoprotective qualities, which could aid in shielding the liver from harm brought on by pollutants or illness.

Even with these possible advantages, licorice root should only be used sparingly because too much of it might have negative consequences like elevated blood pressure, potassium depletion, and hormonal abnormalities. Furthermore, licorice may interact with some drugs, so it's important to speak with a doctor before taking it.

Vidari Kanda

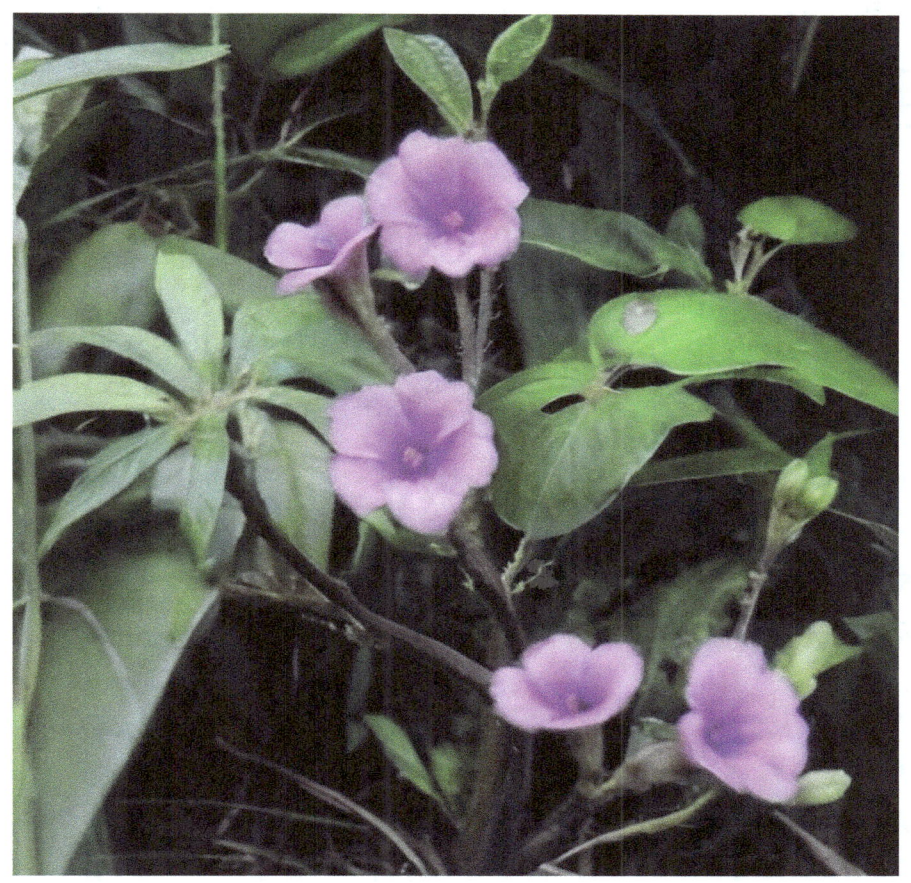

Supports reproductive health.

Native to India, Vidari Kanda is a perennial climbing herb also called Pueraria tuberosa or Indian Kudzu. Because it has so many health benefits, ancient Ayurvedic medicine has employed it. The following are some possible health advantages of Vidari Kanda:

1. Adaptogenic Properties: Vidari Kanda is regarded as an adaptogen, which implies that it could support general wellbeing and assist the body in adjusting to stress.

2. Increases Vitality and Stamina: Vidari Kanda is said to have restorative qualities in Ayurveda, which are said to promote vitality, energy, and stamina.

3. Enhances Libido and Sexual Health: Traditionally used as an aphrodisiac, it is thought to promote both men's and women's sexual health and libido.

4. **Promotes Digestive Health:** Vidari Kanda is believed to improve digestion and ease gastrointestinal problems include bloating, constipation, and indigestion.

5. **Boosts Immune System:** According to certain traditional applications, Vidari Kanda may help the body fend against infections and illnesses by boosting the immune system.

6. **Hormone Balancing:** It is thought to possess hormone-balancing qualities, which could be advantageous for women who are dealing with irregular menstruation or hormonal imbalances.

7. **Effects on Inflammation:** Vidari Kanda has substances that may have anti-inflammatory qualities. These chemicals could help lessen inflammation and ease the symptoms of inflammatory diseases.

8. **Enhances Cognitive Function:** Vidari Kanda's supporters assert that it may benefit brain health and cognitive function, which could lead to an improvement in focus and memory.

9. Promotes Respiratory Health: Vidari Kanda is also used in Ayurveda to promote respiratory health, especially in cases of bronchitis and asthma.

10. Encourages Muscle Growth: Bodybuilders and athletes occasionally use Vidari Kanda to enhance muscle growth and recuperation because of its purported anabolic qualities.

It's crucial to remember that, despite a lengthy history of traditional use and anecdotal data pointing to the herb's health advantages, there hasn't been any scientific research on Vidari Kanda's effectiveness. Before using Vidari Kanda, as with any herbal therapy, it is best to speak with a healthcare provider, particularly if you are on medication or have any underlying medical conditions.

Punarnava

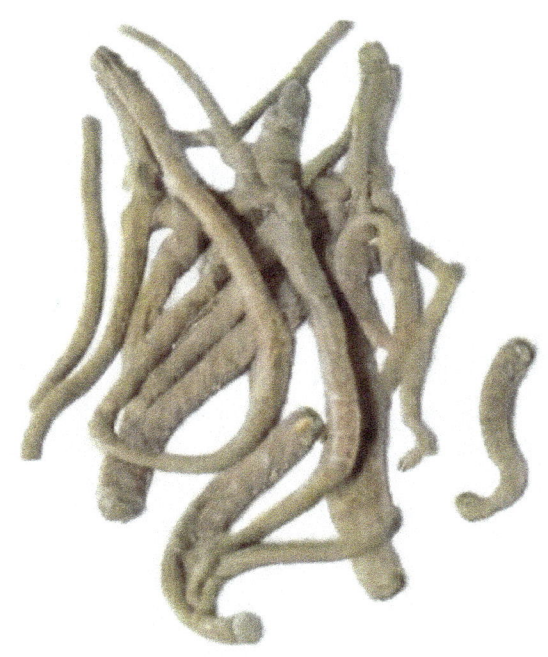

Supports kidney and liver health.

For decades, Punarnava, or Boerhavia diffusa as it is formally named, has been utilized in traditional Ayurvedic therapy. It is widely distributed across the Indian subcontinent and is endemic to India. Punarnava is used to treat a variety of illnesses and is valued for its many health advantages. Here are a few possible health advantages of it:

1. Punarnava is a plant that includes chemicals with anti-inflammatory characteristics. It may be beneficial for ailments including arthritis and inflammatory illnesses since it may help lower inflammation in the body.

2. Punarnava is well-known for having diuretic qualities, which means that it can stimulate the production of urine. This may be helpful when the body retains too much fluid, as in the case of edema.

3. Liver health: Punarnava is believed to have hepatoprotective properties, which means it may help protect the liver from damage. It is used in traditional medicine to support liver health and treat liver disorders.

4. **Kidney health:** Punarnava is frequently used to support kidney health in Ayurvedic medicine. Its diuretic qualities might enhance renal function and facilitate the body's removal of waste.

5. **Cardiovascular health:** Punarnava may have cardioprotective properties, according to certain research. It might assist in lowering cholesterol and blood pressure, which would lessen the risk of cardiovascular illnesses.

6. Punarnava has antioxidants that can assist in scavenging the body of dangerous free radicals. This antioxidant activity may lower the incidence of chronic illnesses and shield cells from harm.

7. Punarnava has been demonstrated to have antibacterial qualities, which suggests that it may be able to combat specific viruses, bacteria, and fungi.

8. **Digestive health:** Punarnava is used in traditional medicine to support digestive health. It may help improve digestion, reduce digestive disturbances, and alleviate symptoms like bloating and gas.

9. Effects against allergies: Research indicates that punarnava may have anti-allergic qualities, which may help to treat respiratory disorders like asthma and allergic responses.

Punarnava has been used traditionally for a variety of health issues and has shown promise in scientific research, but before using it, especially if you have any underlying medical conditions or are taking medication, it is important to speak with a healthcare provider to make sure it is safe and suitable for you.

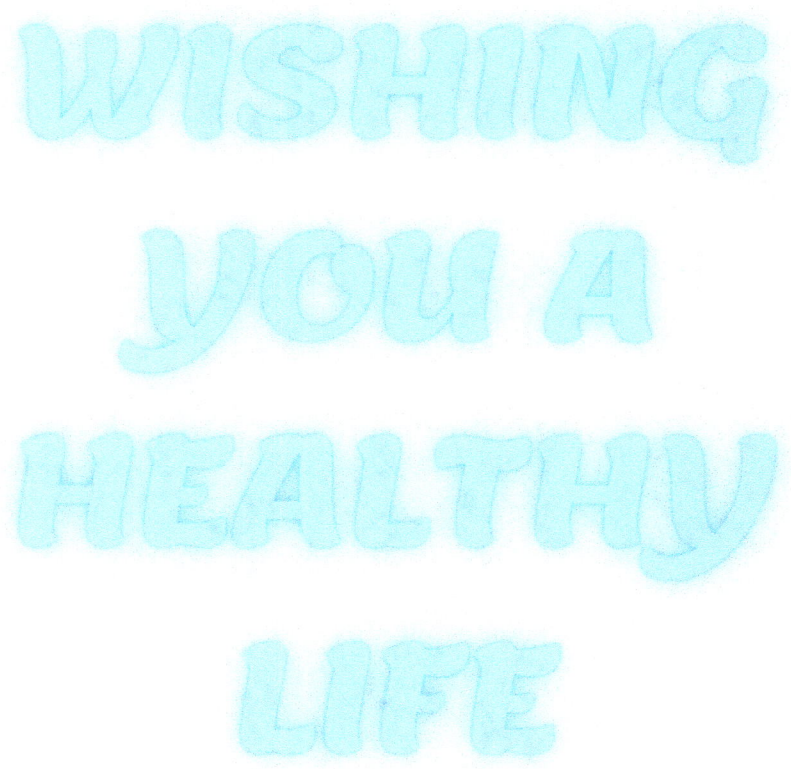

www.ingramcontent.com/pod-product-compliance
Lightning Source LLC
Chambersburg PA
CBHW052151220226
45471CB00004B/1626